IHATOR BROWN PHD

The Mastery Behind Healthy Eating

Explore The Healthy Benefits of Vegetables, Fruits, Meats, Seafood & Grains

First edition

This book was professionally typeset on Reedsy.
Find out more at reedsy.com

Contents

1

Chapter 1: Introduction

D id you know that eating a diet high in fruits and vegetables is beneficial to your health and well-being? Calories from fruits, vegetables, and seafood are lower than those from animal products and processed meals. In addition, it has been shown that increasing your diet of fruits and vegetables lowers your chance of acquiring cancer. A sedentary lifestyle has several disadvantages, and this book discusses them and provides advice on enhancing your diet by including more fruits and vegetables. Consuming foods high in nutrients and antioxidants, such as those found in fruits and vegetables, seafood, and whole grains, may help you feel better and have more energy. These items are essential to maintaining a healthy diet and way of life. There is a great source of vitamins, minerals, and other elements essential for maintaining good health in all individuals. People are becoming more aware of the many health benefits of eating vegetables, fruits, fish, and grains, encouraging them to increase their intake.

If you consume more of these nutrient-dense foods, you will have an easier time avoiding serious health concerns such as diabetes and heart disease. Every day, fresh research highlights the value of ingesting whole, unprocessed foods for our overall health and well-being. However, there has been increasing evidence that nutrients extracted from food may not always deliver the same health benefits as nutrients obtained from their whole food source. Other than commonly recognized nutrients such as vitamins and minerals, phytonutrients and phytochemicals (Phyto meaning "plant") can be found in many plant foods, including herbs and spices, and are particularly beneficial to the health of the body.

Although it was previously believed to be purely a plant benefit, it has since been shown to be an antioxidant that may aid in protecting our cells from the detrimental effects of free radicals and other contaminants. In addition, it has been established that toxins cause DNA damage, and it has also been shown that phytonutrients may help repair that damage and increase communication between cells themselves. Although phytonutrients are unlikely to be required for human survival, their positive health benefits, such as cancer prevention and inflammation reduction, are undeniable and unquestionably contribute to a more enjoyable way of life overall.

According to various scientific studies, eating a nutritious diet from the time we are born and throughout our lives, even our senior years, may significantly influence our overall health and longevity. Eating a well-balanced diet rich in phytonutrients and engaging in regular physical activity might help prevent or postpone the onset of many chronic noncommunicable diseases, such as cardiovascular disease, hypertension, stroke, diabetes, cancer, dental disease, and osteoporosis.

Furthermore, following a healthy diet does not necessitate choosing meal choices based on the amount of fat, cholesterol, sodium, or other nutrients included in the food. While it is true that just because something appears appealing on a nutrition facts label does not imply that it is good for you, it does not imply that the food contained inside it is necessarily nutritious or even useful for you. Whole food diets are associated with lower rates of coronary heart disease, some types of cancer, and other diet-related chronic illnesses. Foods in your diet could be produced from whole grains such as wheat and rye, legumes such as peas and lentils, and nuts and seeds, which are considered nutritious. Cheese and yoghurt are also allowed in the diet, as are small amounts of red meat, fish, chicken, and eggs.

There is no restriction on the amount of dairy consumed. The fact that phytonutrients can only be found in entire plant foods means that a plant-based diet is the healthiest and is also the most pleasurable, making it simpler to maintain a plant-based diet. It's important to be aware of all of the wonderful and exceptional dining alternatives available in each area of cuisine, regardless of where you live, and that is exactly the topic of this book, however, rather than concentrating on what foods to avoid and why this book serves as an introduction or a refresher on what makes excellent cuisine so delicious. To provide the reader with a taste of what each cuisine has to offer, each meal has been described, made, and accompanied by a short history, food chemistry, and nutrition lesson.

According to this definition, food serves as a celebration of the numerous ways it may bring people together around a table, bring cultures together, nourish the body while also nurturing the soul, and make it all possible. The materials and ideas included in each chapter are those that I've learned to be essential to an intuitive method of cooking that is both nutritional and enjoyable. You'll find a multitude of gastronomic pleasures in these pages, all of which I hope will serve as a springboard for the development of your unique connection with food. In addition to being enjoyable, your path of self-discovery will also benefit your health and well-being in various ways. Once you've finished reading the book, it's time to put your fork down and start eating. Investigate your alternatives and enjoy the experience of doing so!

2

Chapter 2: Fundamentals of Healthy Eating

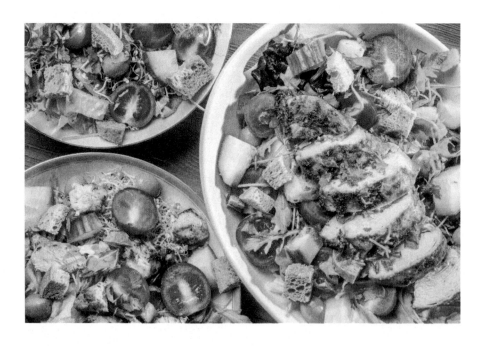

A thorough understanding of nutrition and eating habits and an understanding of how your food affects your mental and physical well-being are required for a well-balanced eating plan. Additionally, eating a healthy diet may aid in weight loss and improve your overall health and wellness. In just a few minutes, you can understand the foundations of a healthy diet, and this information can come in handy if you're attempting to lose weight by medical methods.

The habits of your eating determine the quality of your nutrition. Additionally, several additional elements impact your eating patterns and what you eat and how often you consume it. Instead of a quick fix for weight reduction, a healthy diet is a long-term change in your eating habits that will benefit your long-term health and well-being.

2.1 Healthy diet or anything similar

With each bite of food, your body receives the nutrients, chemicals, and substances it needs to carry out physiological activities such as thinking and metabolism, as well as the energy it requires to function. Foods are an important source of nutrients required for good health and development in children.

Nutrients are available in six different forms:

- Protein
- Carbohydrates
- Vitamins
- Minerals
- Fat
- Water

It is essential to have all six of these nutrients in your diet in order to maintain a healthy weight. A nutritional shortfall occurs when our bodies do not obtain enough of certain nutrients, resulting in the shutting down of our systems. When you don't drink enough water, you run the risk of developing a nutritional shortfall such as dehydration.

2.2 Creating a healthy eating habit

A nutritious diet requires a variety of dietary modifications. As part of this process, you'll need to make certain changes to your diet and eating habits, which will take time. Keep in mind that you should surround yourself with healthy meals when you are attempting to modify your eating habits. Use the following techniques:

- Consumption of complete meals on a regular basis. These are unprocessed, entire foods that are composed mostly of a single ingredient. Healthy foods include fruits, vegetables, meats, nuts, and some grains such as rice, to name a few examples.
- Making the conversion from refined grains to whole grains, refined grains such as sugar and white bread may be replaced with whole grain brown rice and whole wheat bread, respectively. Because of the high fibre content of whole grains, a diet heavy on whole grains is beneficial to your metabolism and digestion.
- It is important to remain hydrated by drinking plenty of water. Water should be consumed in large quantities to stay hydrated and prevent dehydration. Drinking water is the most effective way to combat dehydration since it has neither calories nor sugar. Sugary beverages should be avoided at all costs.
- Instead of concentrating on the foods, you're eliminating from your diet, try to concentrate on the nutrients you're introducing into your system. When it comes to making nutritional adjustments, this may help you stay in a positive frame of mind, which may be beneficial.

Overeating should be avoided at all costs. Adopting healthy eating habits, such as the ones listed below:

- Reduce the number of servings you consume.
- Keeping an eye on the nutrition labels
- Making a conscious effort to avoid overeating due to a habit or mood
- reducing the number of calories consumed

Maintaining a nutritious diet provides several advantages in terms of one's overall health. With a well-balanced diet, the risk of type-2 diabetes and heart disease may be reduced. Another advantage of eating a well-balanced diet is that it helps to keep cholesterol and blood sugar levels in check. In addition to improving your mood and energy levels, eating a balanced diet that is also excellent for your sleep can help you sleep better.

There is no doubt that the great majority of Americans do not consume a nutritionally adequate amount of food. One of the most common causes of weight gain in the United States is a diet high in saturated fat, added sugars, and salt, all of which are consumed in large quantities. As a result, there are 78 million obese adults and 12.5 million obese children in the United States of America.

A healthy diet is one strategy for dealing with this problem. When you live in a world full of diet fads and conflicting nutritional advice, it may be hard to figure out what "healthy eating" means. What does it mean to eat in a healthy way? If you want to get to the bottom of things and learn how to eat more healthy, you've come to the right place. You will learn the information and skills you need to find a diet that will help you live a long and healthy life.

2.3 Eat a healthy diet when travelling

A healthy diet is defined as one that is rich in nutrients and provides you with all of the vitamins, minerals, and energy that you need to maintain your overall health. In order to maintain a healthy diet, one must eat a suitable amount of protein, carbohydrates, and fat, as well as an acceptable amount of fluid. A healthy diet should have a positive impact on both your physical and mental wellbeing.

Each individual's definition of a "healthy diet" will be different, but the following guidelines apply to everyone. This is owing to the fact that each person's dietary needs are different from the next. Depending on their dietary restrictions, some people's ideal diets may look quite different from what you're accustomed to. These restrictions may be based on health, medical, ethical, or religious considerations, among other things. However, while maize and citrus fruits are perfectly acceptable meals for those on other diets, those with GERD should avoid them because they may cause acid reflux in those who suffer from the condition. There are techniques and recommendations in this book that will help you get started on the path to a healthier lifestyle, no matter what your nutritional requirements are.

2.4 Master the art of preparing your own food

Cooking your own food is the best way to ensure that you know exactly what you're putting into your stomach. When you have complete control over what goes into your meals, it is much simpler to exclude harmful ingredients such as added sugars or salt. It is very important that you make your own food to avoid unpleasant side effects that can come from dietary restrictions, especially if you are trying to cut back on certain foods that make your symptoms worse.

As an alternative, you may choose to focus on healthy eating by adding fresh fruits and vegetables as well as lean meats and herbs and spices that are tasty.

By making the switch, you'll have more energy, a healthier body, and, most importantly, better-tasting food.

2.5 Avoid eating processed food

Processing foods should be avoided in accordance with the previously mentioned guidelines. Processing includes the mechanical or chemical altering of a food's flavour or preservation, among other things. Preservatives used in processed foods may have negative effects on the human body, and this is usually done at the expense of the customer. Processed foods include the following items as examples:

- Food that has been canned or frozen
- Biscuits and cookies are baked goods.
- Snacks, both sweet and salty
- Potato chips are a kind of snack food.
- Granola and nut bars are a delicious treat.
- Margarine;
- Ramen noodles; ramen in a can
- soda;

There isn't a difference in the types of quick meals you receive. These processed meals are simply a tiny sampling of the many different types of processed foods that are available at supermarkets. Some of the most prevalent negative effects of these products include acid reflux and other health concerns. They are popular in the American and UK diet, but if you are serious about altering you're eating habits, it is time to eliminate them from your diet completely.

2.6 Pay attention to the nutritional information

Check your diet before you sit down to dinner to be sure you're getting enough nutrients. When you go grocery shopping, be careful since preservatives and added sugar might be found in even the most seemingly innocent of items. When looking at nutrition labels, keep the following rules in mind:

- Unless you pay attention to the serving size, you might be ingesting far more calories, sugar, and salt than you should be. Because the serving size doesn't mean that this is the ideal amount to eat, but rather what the average customer would eat, it's important to remember that.
- While reading the ingredients list, keep an eye out for the daily recommended intake (DV) for each component in the product. This proportion is based on a 2,000-calorie diet; therefore, your actual calorie requirements may differ slightly from these figures.
- Saturated fats, salt, and added sugars are the three most important components to keep an eye out for a while shopping for nutritious meals. As previously mentioned, excessive usage is detrimental to one's overall health.
- Make a list of any items that you do not want to be included in your meal. This is especially important for those who have dietary restrictions.

2.7 Consume natural foods as part of your diet

Despite the fact that the anti-carb craze is growing, carbohydrates are an important part of your diet since they provide your body with the energy it requires. It is vital to understand the difference between healthy and bad carbs. A clean diet necessitates the consumption of entire foods since it enables you to focus on what is beneficial to your health rather than on what is detrimental to it.

2.8 Carbohydrates that are beneficial to your health

Compared to fresh produce, refined meals have been exposed to a great deal of processing. These foods provide all of the fibre and minerals that may be found in naturally occurring foods. Only a few examples include vegetables and fruits in their full form, as well as whole grains and legumes. In contrast to refined carbs, these meals do not produce significant increases in blood sugar levels and hence do not cause you to feel sluggish or weary after eating them. This is especially important to remember for those who have long-term health concerns, such as diabetes.

2.9 Maintaining a nutritional diet plan

When you're just getting started with healthy eating habits, it might be tempting to overindulge in one or two healthy favourites. However, in order to meet all of your nutritional needs, you must consume a variety of foods in a well-balanced meal. Diets high in micronutrients yet low in fat and sugar are regarded as balanced diets. You should include fresh fruits and vegetables, whole grains, and lean protein sources in a healthy diet. Ignoring deficiencies in essential nutrients may result in chronic health problems such as heart disease and cancer in the future if any of these factors are not addressed.

2.10 Sugar, salt, and fat: Consume the bare minimum

We cannot emphasize enough how important it is to keep your consumption of fat, salt, and sugar under control. This ingredient is often found in processed meals. When ingested in large quantities, they may be hazardous. Items containing these substances should be avoided at all costs since they have the potential to derail an otherwise healthy diet.

2.11 Essential fatty acids dietary supplement

Fats have been demonized in the same manner that carbohydrates have been. To maintain a balanced diet, it is important to include a broad range of foods high in healthy fats, such as avocados, nuts, and seeds. Avocados, whole eggs, and different nuts are just a few examples of what you may eat.

2.12 Snacks that are beneficial to your health

Even while processed meals are affordable and widely accessible, they may be detrimental to your health due to their preparation. When it comes to snacking, though, our need for a quick fix usually takes precedence over our better judgment. When it comes to snacking, it's important to keep track of how much you're eating

3

Chapter 3: Benefits of Healthy Eating

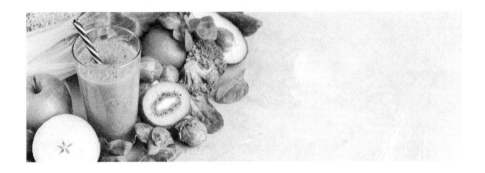

The first step toward a healthy diet is being conscious of what you are eating. We've all heard the adage "you are what you eat" repeatedly and with good reason. Many people, however, find it difficult to change their eating habits because of their hectic schedules or a lack of understanding about the health benefits of eating a well-balanced diet, among other reasons. What does it mean to eat healthily, and what are the benefits of doing so regularly?

What are the benefits of eating healthy? Consuming a diverse selection of foods from the food pyramid is important for maintaining a balanced diet. We may see a considerable improvement in our health if we consume the appropriate amounts of each food group without going overboard. Our health may be improved by increasing our consumption of fresh fruits and vegetables and seafood, carbohydrates, and fibre-rich meals. On the one hand, foods heavy in sugar, salt, fat, and preservatives must be avoided; on the other hand, they must be restricted. The consumption of a well-balanced diet will be to our advantage. An overall healthy diet not only helps our health but also has a positive impact on our whole way of life, bringing more vibrancy and richness into our days. The following are only a few of the most important benefits of eating a nutritious diet:

3.1 The ultimate objective is to lose weight

One of the most important benefits of following a balanced diet is reducing the risk of heart disease. In addition, maintaining a low-calorie diet and avoiding high-calorie choices such as fast food and drinks may help you lose weight. Several fad diets are available, but only a well-balanced diet combined with regular exercise can allow you to lose weight healthily. By incorporating fewer fatty, sugary, and salty foods into your diet, healthy eating guarantees that you get the needed nutrients while maintaining a healthy weight and body composition. Discovering that making small, progressive modifications to your diet will be the most successful technique for maintaining a healthy weight over the long run will be a nice surprise.

3.2 Increasing degrees of dynamism

Your body will thrive on a diet high in protein and carbohydrates, which will keep you energized throughout the day. Breakfast is one of the most important meals of the day and must be consumed as part of a well-balanced diet to be effective. Your ability to pay attention and concentrate throughout the day will improve with time, allowing you to be more productive at work and in your personal life. Become more energetic and avoid the sluggishness of consuming fast food or salty snacks.

3.3 Improve your sleeping patterns

People who eat fast food regularly are more prone to suffering from this condition than others. You may not be aware of it, but your poor eating habits contribute to your high-stress levels, making it harder for you to get a good night's sleep. A nutritious diet improves your body's capacity to cope with stress and prevent hormonal imbalance, which helps it function more efficiently. Practising this will help you deal with the stress of everyday life and teach your body to stay calm and relaxed even when faced with unpleasant or difficult events or situations.

3.4 to live a long and healthy life

Adopting healthy eating habits can help to increase your body's capacity to fight off illness. Fruits and vegetables include a high concentration of antioxidants, vitamins, and minerals, all of which our bodies need to function properly. Consume foods rich in antioxidants to fight the detrimental effects of free radicals. By eating less fat and sugar, you may reduce your risk of getting heart disease, diabetes, and other chronic illnesses.

3.5 Dazzling appearances

Another well-documented effect of eating a balanced diet is the reduction of cholesterol levels. According to the research, people who eat more fruits and vegetables daily tend to look more youthful. Dietary habits that include plenty of fruits and vegetables, meals high in vitamins and minerals, and enough water are essential for living a long and healthy life. Dietary habits such as eating regularly and drinking enough water are the most effective ways to keep the skin looking young and healthy.

3.6 Having a positive attitude about life

Depression has been connected to malnutrition in the past. When you're feeling sad, foods high in B vitamins may be able to help improve your spirits. A well-balanced diet combined with frequent physical activity promotes a positive attitude and a pleasant disposition. Participating in a healthy lifestyle has been shown to boost one's emotional well-being. Healthy, active bodies, enough sleep, and an external appearance that is youthful are all necessary for one to feel positive about one's own person. At the end of the day, health and happiness are inextricably linked.

For many individuals, eating healthy means going on a diet in order to achieve success. This is a common misunderstanding. It is not required to follow a diet in order to get the benefits of a healthy diet. A healthy diet and way of life need long-term adaptations, which must be maintained on a constant basis to be successful. Eating healthy is easy if you follow a well-balanced diet that is rich in all of the necessary ingredients your body needs for optimal performance. Here are some benefits of eating a healthy diet to consider while deciding whether or not to make changes to your lifestyle and diet.

3.7 The deal about healthy eating

If you maintain a healthy eating routine, you will not need to go on a diet in order to notice these benefits. You must have a well-balanced diet in order to maintain a healthy physique. Eating healthy and improving your mood are two important goals that may be achieved by avoiding heavy meals. Eating a healthy diet does not require you to give up all of your favourite dishes.

A healthy diet decreases your chances of getting certain ailments, such as diabetes and heart disease. When it comes to accomplishing this aim, diet and nutrition are critical factors. Your immune system, as well as your overall well-being and psychological well-being, will benefit from a diet rich in vitamins and minerals. Your medical expenses will be lower, and you will save money over time as a result of fewer doctor visits and prescription administration.

Because of this, your mind will be more productive as a consequence of this. The ability to think clearly and swiftly increases when you eat three healthy meals a day and are not hungry or weak. It is critical to have a well-functioning brain. Good nutrition is beneficial to both your physical and mental health, so eating healthily can help you perform better at school or at your place of employment.

The benefits of eating healthily will make you healthier and stronger than others who are not aware of these advantages. In the office or at school, being physically and intellectually strong may give you an edge over your competitors, and it can do ordinary duties at home simpler.

It is expected that improved interpersonal relationships will arise as a consequence of this. Eating healthily will enhance your health and well-being, which will, in turn, improve your interpersonal relationships at home, school, and work, as well as your productivity. As a consequence, your social life will be more enjoyable. As a result of your better demeanour and demeanour, you may even get a raise from your boss. A variety of positive outcomes may be obtained by just being happy and more pleased with oneself. When your mental, physical, and social health is better down the road, you should eat a well-balanced meal plan.

In order to get the full benefits of a well-balanced diet, it is necessary to engage in regular physical activity or sports. When it comes to eating healthy, the essential thing to remember is to eat in moderation. All of your favourite meals may be eaten in moderation if you follow these guidelines.

17

Reduce the portion size of your favourite meals to aid in your weight loss efforts. Aside from that, seek more nutritious alternatives to the things you're already consuming. It should not be necessary to give up your favourite meals in order to gain the advantages of a balanced diet. The meals that you like do not have to make you feel as if you are missing out. Keep an eye on what you eat and how much you consume.

4

Chapter 4: Healthy Eating Plan

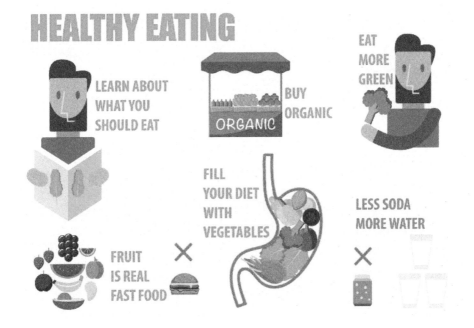

As the prevalence of sickness and obesity continues to rise, an increasing number of people are becoming concerned about their weight and health. Many different diets and weight-loss strategies have been created over the years to help people lose weight in a safe and effective manner while maintaining their health. What it means to be healthy is to be in a state of physical and mental well-being in which all of your body's systems are functioning in harmony with one another. If you want to lose weight, you should follow a diet that delivers all of the nutrients your body requires without exceeding your daily calorie limit. Making a haphazard decision about your food will not provide the desired outcome.

As an alternative, you may be able to attain your optimum level of fitness by making small changes to your diet and adopting a more active lifestyle. Eating a nutritious, well-balanced diet that contains foods from all food groups in the appropriate amounts is essential for good health. It is essential to take your body type and food preferences into consideration while creating a healthy eating plan for yourself. A starvation diet is not essential in order to lose weight or improve your health while following a healthy eating plan as long as you are committed to it. While it may seem that you are being denied, the message is really about sharing your food fairly. In order to maintain a healthy diet, one must eat and drink in line with set rules.

4.1 Steps to help you maintain a healthy diet

The key to maintaining a healthy diet is to make better food choices. The key to maintaining a healthy diet is to do just that: make better food choices. A well-balanced diet includes complex carbs, low-fat fats, and lean protein, all of which contribute to overall health. Make the switch to dairy products that are lower in calories and fat. There are some people who believe that all fats are dangerous fats, which has been a common myth for many decades. This is completely false. Fatty foods are necessary for human life, but they must be the right kinds of fat.

The most prevalent misunderstanding about weight loss is the belief that being overweight is caused by a build-up of fat in the body. In actuality, a range of fats is among the most beneficial foods you can eat for your overall health and wellbeing. In actuality, the right kind of fat may aid in the burning of resistant flab, such as belly fat. In addition, keep an eye on your eating habits and exercise routine. As an added benefit, slowing down your meals may assist you in losing weight and improving your digestive health. Eat slowly so that you can get a better sense of when you are satisfied and when it is time to stop eating.

4.2 Foods that are more nutritious

A gradual approach to making the transition from an unhealthy to a nutritious diet is more beneficial than a quick one. It is well-known that processed foods, frozen dinners, and sugar-sweetened drinks may all be harmful to one's health. Trans fats, salt, artificial sweeteners, and preservatives are abundant in these products, which are made from trans fats that are industrially generated in large quantities. Including natural foods in your diet is important, and fruits and vegetables are excellent choices. Fruits and vegetables are rich in vitamins, minerals, and antioxidants, all of which are essential for good health. Aside from supplying the body with important minerals and fibre, colourful foods provide a delicious and healthy mid-meal snack that is also high in nutrients.

4.3 Reduce your eating portions

It's vital to remember that eating healthy doesn't require a complete ban on all non-healthy foods and beverages. Avoiding a favourite meal just serves to increase your desire for it, and you finally succumb to the temptation. First, reduce the size of your meals, followed by a reduction in the frequency with which you consume them. Healthy cooking techniques such as grilling or steaming, roasting or boiling must be used in conjunction with improved food choices if we are to achieve our nutritional goals. This is a decent rule of thumb to follow in order to avoid losing any nutrients or gaining any additional weight:

4.4 Purify your entire body

The process of detoxification of the body is essential for maintaining good health. When it comes to detoxification, extensive periods of fasting are often associated with the process. However, this is not always the case. Excessive waste has been collected in the body, and detoxification is the method utilized to remove it. A detox diet may be able to assist you in eliminating the toxins that have accumulated in your body as a consequence of bad eating habits and manipulated food. A "detox diet," which is composed entirely of natural ingredients and low in calories, is intended to eliminate waste and restore balance to the body.

It is possible to reduce the number of hazardous chemicals consumed and absorbed from processed foods by following a detox diet on a regular basis. Additionally, it provides healthy meals that promote optimum organ function by providing all of the nutrients necessary for efficient digestion and absorption. When you cleanse your body, you will experience an improvement in both your mental and physical well-being.

4.5 Learn the essentials of healthy eating

Incorporating a healthy eating plan into your lifestyle should not leave you feeling deprived of your favourite foods or as if you have no control over what you consume. It is all about making you happy and healthier when you follow a healthy eating plan! If you pursue the right path, you'll be happier, more confident, and able to recapture the energy that has been lacking in your life. It is possible to achieve all of these goals by following a healthy diet and following the recommendations in your healthy eating guide.

Dieting for better health is the first step on your journey to better health. In terms of nutrition, it is not just about what you eat but also about how much you consume. Healthy eating may help you lose weight, prevent diabetes, and prevent heart disease.

- Heart inflammation is a medical condition that occurs when the heart muscle becomes inflamed.
- A malignant condition that has developed
- Diabetes is a disease that affects the body's insulin production.
- Anxiety's
- There's much more to it!

Additionally, in addition to avoiding these and many other diseases, a healthy eating plan may boost your energy level, help you avoid mood swings, and aid in your memory recall, among other benefits. You may be able to get all of these benefits just by consuming the appropriate meals!

The most important step in developing a healthy eating plan is putting yourself in a position of success. Many people are enthusiastic about the benefits of eating a healthy diet but often fail to take the required measures to ensure that it is a success. To begin with, it's ideal for making things as simple as possible. Contrary to popular belief, starting a diet by calculating calories or weighing your portions can be overwhelming and result in a less healthy diet.

Make a conscious effort to consume a diverse selection of meals that are both aesthetically appealing and nutritionally sound. Consume healthy meals that you like and experiment with different methods to cook them. In no time at all, you'll have tailored your healthy eating plan to fit your own preferences better.

It's not as difficult as it seems to customize a healthy eating plan to meet your own needs and interests. Put your healthy eating guide up slowly and gradually rather than trying to make many adjustments in a short amount of time. Making little effort toward your weight-loss goals can result in positive results and successes that you will be proud of.

Even the tiniest modifications to your healthy eating plan may have a positive impact on your overall health. Setting goals is an excellent way to keep track of your progress, and it's also an excellent way to raise your spirits when you're going through a difficult time. Healthy eating plans are not difficult to develop, and they will have a long-term positive influence on your health and well-being.

When we follow most diets, we end up feeling hungry. Everything seems to be in short supply for you, and you're always concerned about what you could be missing out on. We should avoid attempting to reduce weight in this manner. We end up gaining weight rather than losing weight as a consequence of this detour from our healthy eating regimen. What we need is a well-balanced diet that provides us with satisfaction while also making us feel good about ourselves. These tips can assist you in maintaining your healthy lifestyle.

Meals should not be skipped unless you are following a healthy eating plan that permits you to replace one meal with something nutritious like a smoothie or a snack bar. It is difficult for your body and mind to function properly when you have not eaten for a lengthy period of time. More than anything, you'll be enticed to eat more nutritious items rather than fewer unhealthy ones. Every few hours, consume little portions of food that are satisfying and utilize that meal as fuel for your daily activities. On your healthy eating plan, you will be allowed to eat until you are completely satisfied.

Your healthy eating plan may include a variety of flavours, scents, and textures to satisfy your cravings. It is possible to keep on track with your healthy eating objectives if you plan and prepare your meals in advance. Having regular meals and not having to "grab anything" to eat while on the go reduces our chances of straying from our diets. Bringing a healthy snack with you if you're going to be out of your home for a long amount of time is a good idea.

Bring a list with you to the shop and follow it to the letter. Your healthy eating plan provides you with the opportunity to be creative while preparing tasty and nutritious meals for yourself and your family. Don't take just what looks to be outstanding at the store, and don't spend your time looking around. You'll most likely come to regret your decision in the future. The fact that you are hungry will only increase your cravings and your desire to make impulsive purchases when you get to the market.

Healthy eating plans need the support of others in order to be successful. Nevertheless, attempting to do it on your own may put you at risk of failing miserably in the long run. To execute this job, enlist the help of a close friend, spouse or partner, or a colleague who can provide a hand. This network of individuals who care about you will act as a sounding board and a source of accountability for you throughout your life. If your spouse is equally committed to a healthy lifestyle, this is an excellent way to support one another. Plan your meals, go grocery shopping with your partner, have dinner together, and go to the gym together. It's not a terrible idea to engage in some friendly rivalry from time to time.

It may be pretty irritating to see the same number on the scale day after day after day. A healthy diet and exercise plan should allow you to lose one or two pounds every week if you follow it religiously. As a result, you should weigh yourself once or twice a week or every two weeks at the absolute minimum. Continue to follow your healthy eating plan for another week as a reward for sticking with it throughout the week.

Chapter 5: Healthy Eating Tips & Tricks

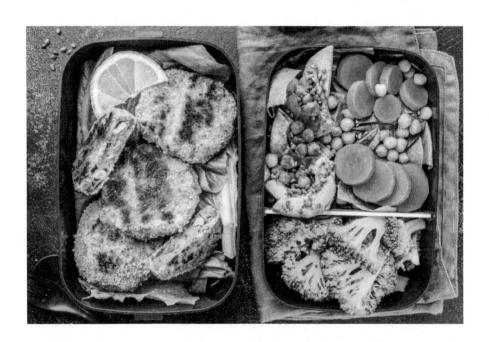

Ahealthy eating routine does not need the use of a set of rigid, uncompromising, flavourless recipes in order to be established. The good news is that you don't have to deprive yourself to the point of fatigue in order to lose weight. Contrary to common belief, it is all about feeling great, having limitless energy, sleeping quietly at night, and being healthy in order to achieve success. It all boils down to minimizing your chance of developing diseases that are often connected with ageing. It's easy to do all of this by slowly transitioning to a simple, healthy eating plan. Continue on your current diet without making a complete 180-degree turnaround.

The most effective method of achieving this goal is via a gradual, step-by-step transition to healthy meal planning. If you're ready to make small, manageable adjustments, you'll be eating more healthy in no time.

Instead of stressing about calorie counts and portion sizes, concentrate on introducing more bright, healthful foods into your diet as a healthy alternative. Recipes requiring the use of fresh fruits and vegetables should be sought out and followed. Your diet will progressively improve in both health and taste as time goes on.

It is important to remember that this is a gradual process rather than an abrupt one. For a few weeks, try adding a bright vegetable salad to one of your daily meals and see how it goes. After that, maybe some fresh fruit can be served as a dessert. Gradually get used to your new position.

The importance of each dietary alteration cannot be overstated. Not all of your favourite foods have to be eliminated from your diet if you want to lose weight quickly and effectively. At the end of the day, you want to feel well, have energy, and reduce your chances of acquiring diabetes, heart disease, or cancer throughout your lifetime.

5.1 Drink plenty of water and exercise

Your body necessitates the consumption of clean, pure water. There is no such thing as "fruit juice" (unless it is freshly squeezed) or "coffee" in the Philippines. Drinking just coffee or very little water may cause dehydration, which is a concern for a large percentage of the population. Your digestive system, as well as all of the organs in your body, needs much water in order to function effectively. In addition to the sugar, flavours, and preservatives in this "fruit juice," your body is unable to break down this "fruit juice"; therefore, it is deposited as fat in your body. Dehydration is the most common side effect of drinking coffee, which is a highly addictive chemical that has a number of negative effects. Coffee is the most widely used narcotic drug in the world.

It's also worth noting that the human body was created for activity rather than the sedentary lifestyle that the majority of people today lead. No matter how little, it's crucial to include a fun activity in your daily routine, even if it's just once or twice a day.

5.2 The key to success is moderation

When it comes to eating a balanced diet, moderation is essential. Your body needs a range of nutrients in order to operate effectively. These nutrients include a variety of carbohydrates, proteins, lipids, and fibre, among others. Smaller portions and less frequent use of some meals are not prohibited.

5.3 Consumption of food

The manner in which you eat is just as significant as the food you consume. When you think of food, you should think of it as a source of nourishment rather than something to be devoured in a rushed way as you race from point A to point B. Breakfast should be had as well. Exercise to get your heart rate up and your lungs expanding in the morning, followed by a light, healthy lunch to start your day off well. Your body craves both physical exercise and nutrition at the same time. After going without food for a long time, your organs are in desperate need of recharging in order to work well.

5.4 "Color is the most important thing."

A diet rich in fruits and vegetables is the key to maintaining a healthy weight. They include a high concentration of minerals, vitamins, and antioxidants. But, to be fair to you, I'm not a great fan of theirs either. Taking little steps toward boosting your diet of fresh vegetables can help you reach your goal. It won't be long before you start to like vegetables because your body wants and needs them.

5.5 Green vegetables

Green vegetables, in addition to the minerals and vitamins they provide (such as calcium and magnesium), as well as the antioxidants they contain (such as vitamins A, C, E, and K), help to boost the circulatory and respiratory systems. Sweet vegetables are an excellent way to satisfy your sweet craving. Cucumbers, carrots, beets, sweet potatoes (also known as yams), winter squash, and onions are all examples of sweet vegetables. Fruit is an essential component of a well-balanced diet. Citrus fruits are rich in vitamin C, while berries are known to be cancer-fighting, and apples are a good source of dietary fibre.

5.6 Consume carbohydrates that are nutritious

Carbohydrates are often referred to as bread, potatoes, pasta, and rice. True, they include carbohydrates, but they are poor carbohydrates—starchy, sugary carbohydrates. You will have erratic blood sugar and insulin levels as a consequence of this due to the rapid breakdown of these carbohydrates into glucose. Carbohydrates may be found in a variety of foods, including fruits, vegetables, and whole-grain products. Remember that I used the term "whole wheat grains" rather than "whole wheat bread" in this sentence.

5.7 Choosing healthy fats over unhealthy fats

Despite the fact that fats are an important part of your diet, there are good and harmful fats to choose from. A suitable quantity of good fat is required for the maintenance of a healthy brain, heart, and other body components (such as hair, skin, and nails). It is critical to include fatty fish such as salmon, herring, mackerel, and sardines in your diet. You must remove trans and saturated fats from your diet in order to maintain a healthy weight.

5.8 Protein

Protein offers the amino acids we need to build muscle tissue and boost our immune system, heart, and respiratory systems, as well as the digestive system. Protein is also important for our overall health. The consumption of protein helps to keep blood sugar levels under control. Red meat is a healthy source of protein in general, and it is especially true for women. Fresh fish such as salmon and other types of fresh seafood, as well as turkey, are fantastic sources of protein that you can include in your diet.

5.9 Calcium for a properly functioning body

Dairy products are, of course, the most apparent source of calcium in the diet. The fact that leafy greens are a fantastic source of calcium should not be overlooked as well. Beans are also a good source of calcium.

5.10 Sodium and glucose

Sugar and salt are required by our bodies, but they must be ingested in moderation. Almost all of today's processed foods are loaded with sugar and salt. Trans fats may be found in a variety of foods, including soy sauce, ketchup, margarine, and instant mashed potatoes, to name a few. If you want a smooth shift, start by progressively eliminating these foods from your eating plan.

5.11 Prepare your meals ahead of time

Make a plan for your meals for the week or the month. The temptation to go for something fast and handy but unhealthy is reduced when meals are prepared ahead of time.

Healthy eating does not need to be a time-consuming and boring diet. The benefits of doing so include improved endurance, improved sleeping patterns, and a lower chance of developing diseases such as diabetes, heart disease, cancer, and other conditions that are mistakenly associated with advancing years of age. Maintain a steady rate of change, and you'll soon find yourself looking forward to more nutritious meal choices.

Despite your best efforts, there is a chance that you may never be able to maintain a healthy weight for your body type. When you start a new diet, you lose a few pounds but then gain them all back. It may be really disheartening. When you keep failing, no matter how hard you try, it's easy to become dissatisfied with your situation. This is a terrible situation.

There is a way out of this sticky situation. Because it does not need hazardous medications, expensive food, or hunger signals, your body will naturally gravitate toward its optimal weight over time.

6

Chapter 6: The Healthiest Fruits

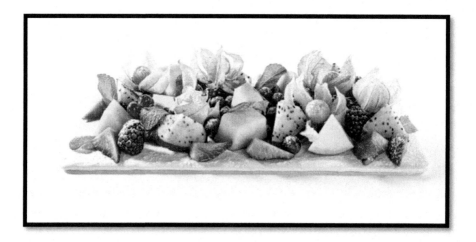

D
ietary fruits are crucial for maintaining and improving overall health and well-being. Sixty per cent of Americans do not consume enough fruits and vegetables. Many people remark that it is tough to fit them in and that it is difficult to fulfil their goals. To meet your daily fruit requirement, you must eat 2 to 3 cups of fruit on average. This will be quite tough for many individuals to cope with. Knowing how to include fruits in your diet, as well as the role they play in achieving maximum health, may serve as an incentive to prioritize them as a component of a healthy

lifestyle choice. Fruits are delicious and bright, and they may be consumed at any time of day. Fruits are low in calories and high in nutrients such as vitamins, minerals, phytochemicals, fibre, and water. In addition, fruits are low in fat and cholesterol. Despite the fact that certain fruits are seasonal, fresh fruits are available at the grocery store all year long, even when local farm output has decreased.

It is important to keep an eye out for food manufacturers that use only small amounts of "genuine fruits" in their goods and mark them as such. A slice of fruit has no health advantages, and claims about the benefits of eating a whole fruit do not apply. Observe the nutritional facts label for a list of the components in the product. Consider if the words "whole fruit" or "fruit flavoured" are included among the ingredients. If something is "fruit flavoured," it does not qualify as a fruit.

The majority of fresh fruits have tastes that are either sweet or tart. Low-calorie, high-nutrient meals are often more appealing than high-calorie, low-nutrient foods, and they are often more nutrient-dense. Pure fruit refers to dried, canned, or frozen fruits that have not been sweetened or flavoured in any manner, shape, or form. By including a variety of fruits in your diet, you can ensure that you are getting a variety of vitamins and minerals. Examples of fruits that are high in vitamin C include berries, bananas, fibre and vitamin-A-rich mangoes. Consume a wide range of fruits on a daily basis. Eaten in large amounts, a wide range of nutrients and health benefits can be found in a wide range of fruits.

Dry fruits such as raisins, cranberries, and prunes should be consumed in moderation since the drying process increases their calorie content. A cup of fresh grapes has around 104 calories, and half a cup of dried cranberries contains approximately 220 calories. Another option is to consume freeze-dried fruits, which are low in calories, delicious, and keep practically all of their nutrients when consumed. They are, on the other hand, rather expensive.

A serving of fruit contains 100 per cent of the fruit's juice. The full fruit of orange, on the other hand, has just 62 calories and 3 grams of fibre. Even though a half-cup amount of juice, including the pulp, has the same number of calories as a whole orange, the absence of fibre is the most significant difference.

6.1 The worth of a yoghurt

Fruit is often included in yoghurt. Because of the small amount of fruit in the recipe, increasing the sugar content increases the calorie count. Plain low-fat yoghurt is better than full-fat yoghurt because you can add your own fruit to it.

5.2 The science behind fruits

Fruits are beneficial to your cardiovascular health, and you should consume lots of them. Women in Finland have been proven to benefit from including 12-cup (4-ounce) portions of the following fruits and berries in their daily diets by blending and pureeing them. After eight weeks, their HDL (high-density lipoprotein) cholesterol level had increased by 5.2%. Long-term consumption of fruits has been associated with a lower risk of developing cancer. When more than 42,000 Japanese people were polled, it was shown that those who consumed citrus had a decreased chance of developing all types of cancer. A wide range of factors might have an impact on the outcome of the experiment. According to one theory, the flavonoids found in lemons may have the ability to delay the formation of cancer cells. Especially when it comes to weight loss, fruits are a priceless source of nutrition.

Researchers in Brazil ran a trial in which they urged women to eat three apples, pears, or an equal number of fibre-rich oat biscuits each day to lose weight. Over the course of the study's ten weeks, fruit eaters lost about 2 pounds, but oat eaters maintained their weight, the researchers found. Fruits are a great snack or complement to your three daily meals because of the fibre and nutrients they provide. It's important to remember that "sweetness" and "acidity" are both subjective sensations. Fruit eaten before the peak season may have a greater acidity level than fruit ingested during the peak season. Fruit consumed before or after its peak season may have a less acidic or sweeter flavour than fruit consumed during its peak season. Fruits that are mealy or pithy may be found at the end of the season, with little flavour left.

6.3 Fruits and vegetables on the international stage

Make fruits a significant component of your daily diet. Choose from a variety of fruits that are brightly coloured, tasty, and high in nutrients. Sweet and savoury meals that we like include antioxidant-rich fruits such as blueberries and strawberries, citrus fruits and apricots, kiwifruit, cantaloupes and watermelons, as well as apples and pomegranates, among other fruits and vegetables. Fresh, cooked chutneys for grilled meats, poultry, and fish and salads topped with them are just a few of the ways to prepare and enjoy these fruits of the earth. Look at the exotic fruits at your local supermarket next time you go grocery shopping. They come from all over the world and have been brought to us by a variety of technologies and transportation methods.

There are alternatives for fresh, frozen, and tinned produce. You may purchase them in the same manner as our native fruits: fresh, frozen, tinned, or dried, depending on your preference. We should not take for granted the availability of these fruits since they come from all over the globe and are not always in season. The most important sources of these fruits are kiwis from New Zealand and mangoes from India or the Caribbean. Despite their age, these berries are in excellent shape with no evidence of damage. You may want to include them in your fruit-picking excursion if possible. You're doing a favour for your body and your health by doing this. Given that you've read this book, you're probably aware of how important fruits are to our health and well-being. As a result, include fruits in your everyday diet. You're also aware of how tasty fruits are and how they keep our taste buds pleased.

5.4 Utilizing fruits to their full potential

Fruits are nature's candies, and they may be found in plenty all around us. They're not only delicious and freshly picked, but they're also beneficial to your health. They are a fantastic source of energy since they are rich in nutrients such as vitamins, fibre, and enzymes. Fruit, on the other hand, has both good and negative characteristics. When you read this chapter, you'll learn about some of the most common health risks that fruits can cause, as well as how to avoid them.

Today's large-scale fruit agriculture is plagued by chemical and pesticide contamination, which is a major concern. There has been a relationship established between the use of numerous chemicals and infertility, cancer, and other health problems. In addition to being among the most difficult fruits to grow, peaches, grapes, and pears have been discovered to have higher amounts of pesticides than other fruit varieties.

In order to protect ourselves from exposure to dangerous chemicals and pesticides, we should always go for the finest quality products that are available on the market. Organic fruits are more expensive, but the superior quality, taste, and nutritional content more than compensate for the higher price. The best location to get fresh, organic fruits and veggies is at your local farmer's market. As an alternative, you could sign up for an organic food delivery service or start your own organic garden from scratch. Always wash fruits and vegetables well before eating them, and if they are not organic, peel them first.

It is critical that the fruit be eaten as soon as possible once it has been harvested. By serving fruit as an after-dinner dessert, it has the opportunity to mix with high-protein and high-fat meals and linger in the stomach for an extended period of time. Fruit ferments as a result of the raised stomach temperature, in a similar way to how grapes ferment to produce wine. It is easy to feel jittery and buzzed after consuming an excessive amount of fruit after a substantial meal.

Fruit should only be ingested when your stomach is entirely empty in order for it to be digested as soon as possible. Because of this, it is best to consume it on its own. For example, you may have a fruit salad for breakfast or as a snack in between meals to keep you healthy. If you'd like, you can start dinner with a glass of freshly squeezed juice as an appetizer. When you eat, it will be quickly absorbed and will help you not to overeat so that you won't eat too much food.

Fructose is a kind of simple sugar that may be found in fruits and other foods. Fructose, like glucose, is swiftly metabolized by the human body, leaving behind acidic residues in the process. A large amount of fruit causes the stomach and blood to become acidic, resulting in vomiting and diarrhoea. Your body is incapable of coping with an excessive amount of acid. The average Western diet, lack of physical activity, and everyday stress all contribute to the creation of an environment that is both exceedingly toxic and acidic in composition. An acidic environment in the body, along with a lack of alkaline foods in our diet, is thought to be the root cause of many modern illnesses.

To counterbalance the acidity induced by the sugar in fruit, green leafy vegetables, which are rich in alkalinity, may be used as a substitute. You may garnish your fruit salad with a little finely chopped parsley. Incorporate a few delicate lettuce leaves into your fruit or fresh spinach into your fruit juice smoothie for a more substantial flavour. Many of the fruit recipes that I use are based on the notion of balancing the pH and decreasing the acidity of the fruits.

If you eat much fruit and don't undertake much physical activity, the energy you don't consume will be stored as fat in your body. As a result of their high carbohydrate content, sweet fruits with high sugar content, such as grapes, cherries, and ripe bananas, have a high-calorie count. Among the many benefits of fruits is the presence of fibre, which keeps you feeling full for a longer period of time. The absence of fibre in both the juice and certain fruits makes it easy to overindulge in fruit juice, which may lead to weight gain.

Moderation is essential when it comes to eating any meal. The key to losing weight is to consume fewer high-quality meals in greater quantities. A few serving size suggestions are included in the table below: One banana, two little apples, three apricots, one cup of grapes, and one bowl of cherries make up this portion of the meal. Drink just one glass of fruit juice at a time, and be certain that it is natural and made entirely of fruit. If you're thirsty, drink some water.

Sweet fruits have large amounts of acidic sugars, which contribute to the development of dental disease. Because of the nature of bananas, they leave many residues between the teeth, but the peel of grapes gets in the way. Citrus fruits, like oranges and grapefruits, have a lot of acid in them, which can hurt your teeth.

After eating fruit, brush your teeth thoroughly and floss between your teeth to remove any fruit skins that may have been stuck between your teeth while you were eating. Straw should be used for juice consumption, and after eating or drinking fruit, you should rinse your mouth with water to prevent bad breath.

Even though fruits are very healthy and natural foods, it is important to follow the guidelines outlined above in order to avoid negative health consequences. At a reasonable price, you can get the best local, seasonal, and organic fruits, so make your selection carefully. Eaten on an empty stomach, either by themselves or with a side of leafy greens, they are the most flavorful. Maintain a nutritious diet and brush your teeth after every meal.

6.5 Fruits and their health benefits

Fruits, which are among God's most beautiful creations, are also offered to us as a source of nutrition. People have been picking wild fruits for food since the days of Adam and Eve, according to legend. Many people like fruits because of their appearance and taste but often fail to realize how nutritious they may be for their overall health. Fruits are mostly made of simple carbs such as fructose and sucrose, with a little bit of fibre thrown in for good measure. Aside from vitamins A and C, minerals such as potassium, and lesser amounts of other nutrients, the best source of natural sweeteners contains a variety of additional nutrients. We need a diverse spectrum of nutrients, which may be found in fruits, in order to maintain a healthy body. It is certain that fruits, with their sweet and savoury taste combinations, have risen to take a major role in the natural food diet.

When purchasing fruits, it is preferable to choose locally farmed and seasonally available vegetables. Consuming fruits that have a cooling impact on the body is recommended for those who have overheated blood systems. According to traditional Chinese medicine, those who have a cold blood system should avoid consuming cooling fruits since they may cause the wind to be produced. As a consequence of the presence of wind in the body, tremors, convulsions, and other symptoms may develop. Epilepsy, arthritis, and rheumatoid arthritis are among conditions that may be exacerbated by some cooling fruits. It is critical to understand the nature of the fruits from which they are derived, as well as whether they are cooling, neutral, or warming in nature, in order to enjoy the advantages of fruits. The following are some examples of the health benefits that might come from the things you do:

The apple is a pleasant fruit with a taste that is both sweet and acidic. This kind of apple has a mellower taste than the others. Despite the fact that apples contain a small quantity of vitamin C, the vitamin is quickly depleted if the fruit is stored for a lengthy period of time. Apples have a low sodium level but a high potassium content, which helps to strengthen the heart muscle by increasing blood flow. Constipation may be relieved by eating an apple with the peel on it, and eating an apple with the peel on it can aid individuals in recuperating from sickness with their digestion. People with a cold blood system may find that steaming apples helps to lessen the cooling effect of the fruit.

It's difficult to make a bad choice while choosing a date. All of these vitamins and minerals may be found in large quantities in these fruits and vegetables. In terms of nutrition, red dates are beneficial for replenishing fluids and blood, easing diarrhoea, cleaning the internal body, and bringing the mind into balance. Dates are effective in easing and lubricating coughs. For red dates to change into black dates, they must first be dried out in the sun and then steamed before being cooked in an oven. This is repeated again and over again in order to turn them completely black. A little warming effect is felt by the body as a result of their use. Please be advised that an excessive number of dates may cause bloating and the formation of mucus in the digestive tract and throat.

Kiwi fruits are a combination of sweetness and sourness, and they have a cooling impact on the body. These meals are high in vitamin C, fibre, and magnesium, all of which are essential nutrients. Phytonutrients assist in the repair and growth of bones and teeth, as well as the reduction of blood pressure and cholesterol levels, as well as the improvement of the structure of the blood vessels. When choosing kiwi fruits, you should opt for ones that are firm yet give slightly when you press on them. The finest way to use it is with a chilled, simple teaspoonful scooped just off the skin. When eating kiwi fruits, those who are sensitive to them should be informed that they may suffer from coughing and wheezing as well as other symptoms of an allergic reaction.

Pineapples have a sweet and tart taste that may vary from neutral to warming in temperature. The healthiest pineapples are those that have been allowed to ripen in the sun. The size and intensity of the fragrance, as well as the fullness of the eyes, are all good indicators of the maturity of the fruit. Make sure the fruit's stem isn't withering before eating it. It is not recommended to acquire pineapples that have faded fruit stalks. The warmth provided by pineapples that are sour or underripe is reduced. When you're thirsty, grab a pineapple to quench your thirst. These herbs help to keep the spleen healthy, improve digestion and urine, reduce swelling, and stop diarrhoea by working on the digestive system, which is why they do this.

Star fruits, which are sweet and somewhat astringent, have a cooling to warming impact on the body. In general, green and sour fruits are colder in the wild, but yellow and sweet fruits are warmer in their natural environment. Star fruits also promote the action of the salivary glands, which aid in the production of body fluids. Fever is lessened, and the production of urine is encouraged. There are other benefits to eating star fruits, too. They can help with digestion and stomach problems, lower blood pressure and coughing and throat irritation, and help the body clean itself.

Fruit outperforms all other foods in terms of nutritional content. We may pick from a wide variety of fruit varieties, many of which are abundant in nutrients and beneficial to our overall health. Fruits have a high concentration of vitamins, minerals, and phytochemicals, which is why they are so beneficial to your health. It has also been shown that the most effective method of obtaining the benefits of each vitamin is to eat the fruit or juice as a whole rather than take nutritional supplements.

Fruits, vegetables, greens, and beans are good weight-loss foods because of their low-calorie content, large volume, and high concentration of key nutrients. Fruits, vegetables, greens, and beans are also excellent sources of fibre. On a practical level, they are able to give a significant quantity of energy without consuming a significant amount of fat or calories. When your stomach is stuffed with high-volume, low-calorie meals, there is less room for other items to fit in. Researchers have found that plant-based diets may also help people feel less hungry and stop overeating, according to recent studies.

Fruit's health benefits can only be completely realized if we eat at least five pieces of fruit each day in order to get the most benefit from them. Many people who are attempting to lose weight may also find that eating fruit is beneficial to their efforts. The taste, fibre content, calorie density, and variety of the meal are thought to be the most important factors influencing energy consumption. Some of these difficulties may be alleviated by eating a diet high in fruits. Fruits, in part, may help you lose weight because they have a lot less sodium in them naturally. This may help you lose weight by reducing the amount of water in your body.

The consumption of at least one-third of your daily calories from fruits and vegetables may assist you in losing weight more rapidly since fruits and vegetables fill the stomach more quickly, enabling you to eat fewer high-calorie meals. No matter how much fruit and vegetables we eat, our total calorie consumption will be lower. Despite the fact that it is possible to eat a wide variety of fruits without going over calorie limits, it is more difficult to keep your weight in check.

6.6 Using fruits to help you lose weight

These fruits are great for weight loss because of their high fibre content, low-calorie content, and high concentration of the antioxidant vitamin C. You should eat foods high in vitamin C on a regular basis since vitamin C helps to reduce fat absorption in the body. If you consume many fruits, you may be able to lose a few pounds every week since they are both tasty and low in calories.

Bananas have far more fibre than apples when compared side by side. Apples are excellent because they are even more filling than regular apples, which is amazing. This is owing to the fact that the banana has far more fruit than the apple. The convenience of having a banana on hand while you're on the go is an additional perk of eating one. An unripe banana may be devoured by simply snatching one off the counter and sticking it in your mouth. Simple. A whole banana may be consumed in less than a minute. Bananas are excellent for weight loss for all of the reasons listed above.

There is a multitude of reasons why apples are one of the most effective fruits for losing weight. As a fruit that is high in nutrients, apples are one of the most effective fruits for weight loss. Eat plenty of apples if you want to maintain a healthy and active lifestyle. It has been shown that consuming Vitamin C has a beneficial effect on fat absorption in the body. In addition to the above benefits, apples are among the best fruits for weight loss available for a variety of reasons, including the following:

I'll say it again: fruits with low sugar content and high carbohydrate content are the most effective for weight loss. The reality is that you may lose weight by eating a broad range of fruits, which is something you should do. Fruits are a great way to lose weight for a variety of reasons, including their high fibre content. As a source of fibre, fruits are a fantastic way to reduce weight and keep the pounds off. Increasing the amount of fibre in your diet may assist your digestive system in moving food through your body and out of your system. Fruits that are both satisfying and low in sugar are the best choices for anyone looking to lose weight.

- It may be possible to lose weight.
- improved ability to participate in physical activities
- Heart disease is less likely to occur.
- Cancer development has a lower chance of occurring.

- Reduce the pressure in your arteries.
- It is possible to lower cholesterol levels.
- The likelihood of developing type 2 diabetes is lowered.
- Having the ability to slow down the ageing process
- Fruit may help you lose weight!

A great number of men and women have discovered that eating fruits may help them lose weight, and you're going to become one of those people. Besides providing us with the vitamins and minerals we need to maintain optimum nutrition, fruits and vegetables have been shown to aid in weight loss in certain people. In particular, fruits, which are considered high-sugar foods, are underappreciated, and this is a shame. Yes, fruit does contain sugar, but it is a natural sugar that has not been refined and processed in the same way that sugar found in pastries and ice cream has been. In other words, fruit consumption provides a convenient way to get the vitamins and minerals your body needs while also meeting your daily carbohydrate requirements.

There seems to be a connection between eating fruit and losing weight. Fruits that are high in carbohydrates may be substituted for other carbohydrate-dense meals, such as those that are high in fat and cholesterol, provided they provide a sufficient quantity of carbohydrates. When it comes to a sweet treat, nothing surpasses a single serving of fresh strawberries when it comes to freshness and flavour. Fruits will meet our sugar and carbohydrate requirements, but they will not cause us to gain weight since they do not include any unnecessary additions or preservatives. Therefore, fruits are superior substitutes for refined carbohydrates, and they also include necessary vitamins and minerals. Which fruit, out of all the options available, is the most effective for weight loss?

Because not all fruits are created equal, you may want to be careful with your fruit-eating when it comes to weight loss. Keeping the amount of sugar in your diet as minimal as possible may help you lose weight if you're attempting to get in better shape. As a consequence of this knowledge, you should avoid starchy fruits such as bananas, dates, plantains, and breadfruit. Fruits such as strawberries and apples are ideal examples of non-starchy foods that should be prioritized. In addition to reducing the number of carbohydrates in your diet, you should pick fruits that are high in fibre as your major source of fruit consumption. A few of the numerous berries that are high in fibre are blueberries, blackberries, and raspberries, to name just a few. The following fruits have a high fibre content: kiwis, pears, and apples, among others.

According to a number of sites, grapefruit, all sorts of berries, watermelon, cantaloupe, and peaches are among the most popular fruits for weight loss. In order to use fruit as a weight-loss aid, it is essential that you eat the fruit in its natural condition whenever possible. Fresh fruit does not contain any preservatives, making it a preferable choice over processed or canned fruits in many ways. It is not possible to consume fruit in a pastry and claim to be consuming fruit. When it comes to reducing weight, though, putting blueberries on a cheesecake is a very different kettle of fish.

6.7 Fruit variety health Benefits

In addition to being a fantastic source of vitamins and minerals, antioxidants, phytochemicals, and fibre, fruits also include a variety of other nutrients that are good for your health. Phytochemicals, which are mostly found in plants, may help protect your health. Antioxidants are molecules that protect the body against free radicals, which are harmful to the body's cells. Unlike vegetables, fruits do not contain cholesterol.

- Almost all of the fruit's nutrients come from water, which makes up between 70% and 80% of the fruit's total weight.
- As a result of their inherent sugar content, fruits are easy to consume, and we are all born with a need for sweetness. This dish has a wonderful taste and is a delight to consume. Including them in your diet or way of life isn't difficult in the least.

- What is the proverbial "an apple a day keeps the doctor away"? Have you ever heard of this adage?
- Why not start with one apple a day to see how it goes? I'm not suggesting that you limit yourself to one apple each day. If you want to get the nutritional benefits of fruits, you should consume a variety of fruits on a daily basis.
- Having a piece of fruit before and after lunch, or at the beginning and conclusion of each meal, is perfectly acceptable.
- Also, remember to incorporate fruits into your children's daily meals as well.
- As an extra plus, fruits need no preparation or cooking other than a brief wash before consumption. Remember to keep them refrigerated at all times.
- Fruit should be consumed on a regular basis in order to maintain a healthy diet. During your journey to work, munch on some fruit, such as strawberries, grapes, or small tomatoes, that are easy to eat while you work or watch television, such as a banana or an apple. Sliced fruits may be added to cereal or yoghurt for breakfast, or they can be eaten on their own.
- As an alternative, you may ingest them. Consider yourself fortunate to have the simple joy of juicing!
- When compared to the vegetable component of the experts' 5 A Day recommendation, fruit consumption is a piece of cake. The rationale for this is that you may either juice the fruits and then drink them, or you can just mix the fruits and drink them as a whole.
- You may also add more flavour by juicing the vegetables or combining them with healthy yoghurt.
- Some people believe that eating fruits in their natural state rather than juicing them is better. However, they are true in the sense that when people talk about juicing, they are referring to the process of removing the pulp from a juicer from the fruit. You may utilize the pulp in a variety of ways, like baking a cake or biscuit mix or boiling beans with it while they're cooking! The pulp should be part of your daily diet because it has

the fibre you need from fruit nutrition and should be eaten in moderation.

- As a result, I prefer to use my second juicer, which functions in the same way as a blender, rather than the one that really juices. Before mixing the ingredients, I don't bother to separate the pulp from the rest of the components first. It is true that for some people, a "smooth" smoothie with no pulp is more practical and more appealing than a smoothie with pulp.
- That's OK, as long as you make an attempt to ingest the pulp in some way or another.
- And if you don't currently consume fruits, don't be concerned with the pulp for the time being; just begin to consume fruits as soon as possible. We'll finally come to the point of suffocation. More than half of a piece of fruit is preferable to none at all.
- Fruits have a wide range of vitamins and minerals that help keep your immune system strong.
- They claim that eating five pieces of fruit and vegetables every day will aid in the prevention or treatment of cancer and heart disease, as well as a variety of other lifestyle problems such as diabetes and elevated cholesterol.

6.8 The importance of fruits

Many people prefer to eat meat rather than fruits and vegetables, and this is understandable. When it comes to dessert, most people choose chocolate cake over a fruit bowl, which is understandable. You should, on the other hand, eat more fruit platters if you want to live a healthier lifestyle. Fruits should be included in everyone's diet, regardless of their age or gender. You might be surprised to learn that dieters are often told to eat a lot of fruit.

Why is it that fruits get so much attention when it comes to one's health? In part because of the large variety of fruits that are often seen in a fruit bowl, it is an excellent source of vitamins and minerals. Indulging in fruit platters gives an extra source of fibre, which benefits the cleaning process by encouraging regular bowel movements on a daily basis. Besides supplying more water, fruits may also make you feel fuller, which may reduce your urge to overindulge in unhealthy foods.

If you need a lot of a certain vitamin, you may always pick fruits that are abundant in that vitamin. Choosing orange or yellow fruits, for example, will provide you with more vitamin A than other fruits. For example, peaches and bananas are examples of fruits that are rich in vitamin A, which helps to enhance visual acuity, bone density, and the appearance of the skin. Pears and apples, which are high in vitamin B1, are good sources of this vitamin, as are other brown or white fruits such as apricots, which are also high in vitamin B1. If you're a big lover of Vitamin C, be sure to eat enough strawberries and oranges from fruit platters.

The consumption of raw fruit, as opposed to cooked fruit, is the most efficient method of obtaining the greatest number of vitamins from a fruit. When choosing which fruits to buy, it is best to pick ones that have been recently harvested rather than those that have been harvested a few days earlier.

If you're attempting to lose weight, fruit platters are also a fantastic alternative. It's likely that some people aren't aware of this, but eating fresh fruit on a regular basis may be really beneficial when it comes to weight loss. The reason behind this is that, as compared to other foods, fruits are relatively low in calories. However, due to the high sugar content of grapes and dates, these fruits are not recommended for weight loss since they contain a high amount of carbohydrates and are high in sugar. It is suggested that you nibble on fresh fruit rather than processed meals if you are trying to shed some pounds.

CHAPTER 6: THE HEALTHIEST FRUITS

Chapter 7: Explore the Hidden Powerful Fruits

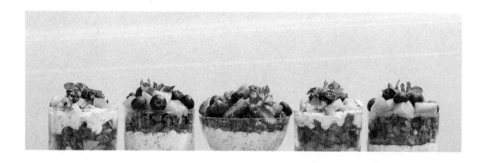

There are numerous plants in the realm of food that many people mistakenly believe are vegetables but which are true fruits in the truest sense. The tomato is, without a doubt, the most well-known of these examples. Ultimately, the Supreme Court was obliged to intervene and settle the argument in 1893, deciding that it should be categorized as a fruit rather than a vegetable when it became too hot to handle. The true problem is with the seeds, not with the sweetness. According to the dictionary, a fruit is "something that grows on a plant and is the means by which that plant sends its seeds out into the world."

For the avoidance of doubt, the fruit is not a component of the plant but rather a reproductive part of the plant. According to the definition, the tomato plant's output, in contrast to the egg that a chicken lays, is not a constituent component of the bird itself. When we consume vegetables, we are, on the other hand, consuming the plant itself or some of its components, such as roots, stems, and leaves. You don't have to eat just tomatoes to be a true fruit. Many other vegetables you eat every day are also fruits.

7.1 Tomatoes

Despite the fact that tomatoes are classified as fruits by the USDA, the majority of people still consider them to be vegetables. The fact that the Supreme Court determined that tomatoes should be taxed with other fruits and vegetables in 1893 was based on this line of reasoning. Justice Horace Gray characterized the argument: The court's opinion found that tomatoes, like cucumbers, squashes, beans, and peas, are "fruits of a vine", according to Gray's definition. However, in the common language of the people, "all of these are vegetables grown in kitchen gardens, and whether eaten cooked or raw, they are typically served at dinner in conjunction with the soup, fish, or meats that constitute the main part of the repast, rather than as a dessert, as is the case with most fruits." Among the vegetables that are really fruits are cucumbers and eggplants, as well as tomatoes and pumpkins, as well as melons and okra, among a variety of other vegetables. For starters, these fruits are referred to as vegetables due to the development of their seeds as well as the fact that they are grown mostly for their blooms.

There are many fruits that will claim to be veggies, no matter whom you ask when they are not. It's doubtful that even inquiring farmers and teachers would supply an explanation, but, since one provides us with food and the other teaches us, we have little option but to keep silent on the issue of both professions. Consequently, we are here to provide you with all of the scientific knowledge you need in order to improve your reasoning skills. Tomatoes are used in our cooking on a daily basis. The vines of a tomato plant may produce fruit in addition to seeds, so classifying it as a fruit since it is a fruit because it is a fruit (tomatoes). Despite the fact that these fruits are often used in cooking, they are still referred to as "vegetables" in many people's thoughts, despite the fact that they are fruits.

If you've ever been perplexed as to whether a tomato is a vegetable or a fruit, you now know how to distinguish the two. Although the tomato is considered a fruit by the general public, botanists consider it strictly a herb. If you plant tomato seeds in any soil, they will sprout and thrive if you supply them with enough water and room. Tomato seeds are very contagious.

7.2 Peppers

According to the USDA, every kind of pepper, from bell peppers to jalapenos, qualifies as a fruit rather than a vegetable. Peppers are not strictly vegetables, despite the fact that the majority of people believe they are. Unlike other plants, peppers contain tiny seeds that mature into fruit after emerging from their flowers. No matter whether you're talking about a jalapeno or bell pepper, they have all been considered fruits in the botanical meaning of the word. Because of its "hot" taste and its Solanaceae origin, it may be used in a variety of culinary applications. For those of you who like spicy food, you've definitely eaten it on a regular basis at some point. It is a fantastic source of nutrition for our bodies since it is high in vitamins C and A, fibre, folic acid, and potassium, among other nutrients. By making the food spicier, it also becomes tastier in the process.

7.3 Pumpkins

Anyone who has ever carved a pumpkin into a jack-o-lantern for Halloween is fully aware of the large number of seeds that are contained inside the fruit. According to the USDA's definition, pumpkins and all other gourds are considered fruits rather than vegetables. The pumpkin, which is most typically associated with Halloween, is loaded with seeds and has a thick interior made up of grains and water, as anybody who has ever cooked with one will tell you.

The pumpkin is also known as a gourd in certain parts of the world. If you want to increase the number of pumpkins you produce, all you have to do is consume the seeds that are within the pumpkin. Cucurbits, which belong to the Cucurbitaceae family, have a lot of vitamins E, C, and iron, as well as other nutrients.

7.4 Cucumbers

Cucumbers are a surprise member of the gourd family, despite their appearance. Were you ever going to look back on pickles with the same fondness as you do now? Cucumber is a low-calorie fruit that is high in antioxidants and anti-inflammatory substances, making it beneficial to our health in many ways. It has been used as a home remedy for skin restoration since it is a good source of nutrients and may assist in keeping your body well-hydrated. In fact, cucumbers are classified as fruits due to the presence of seeds, and if you ever grow cucumbers in your garden, you'll observe that the plant from which they are harvested blossoms. It is in the Cucurbitaceae family, which also contains cucumbers. It is classified as an edible plant, and the majority of its cultivars are edible.

Vegetables that are really fruits are distinguished from vegetables by the fact that they all contain seeds and are derived from flowering plants. Unlike fruits, vegetables often have roots and leaves in addition to seeds. An excellent illustration of this is our cucumber, which has a surprising quantity of seeds despite the fact that the seeds are a valuable source of nutritional fibre and nutrients. Fruit is a plant that blooms with flowers and subsequently produces fruit, but other parts of the plant, such as the stems, roots, and leaves, are referred to as vegetable parts. The fruits of plants contain seeds that may be used to propagate additional flowers, but the roots, stems, and leaves of the plant do not carry any seeds. Only fruits with a high concentration of seeds and a high concentration of water should be ingested. The seeds found in a variety of fruits and vegetables that you eat on a regular basis are easy to find.

7.5 Eggplant

No, it is not a kind of fruit. The eggplant is classified as a berry rather than a fruit, owing to the fact that the seeds are edible. Farmers cultivate it as a member of the Solanaceae family throughout the growing season. The eggplant, which is oval in shape, purple in colour, and derived from flowering plants, is often referred to as an eggplant. The presence of seeds, on the other hand, would elevate it even farther into the category of fruit, given that it is a fruit rather than a vegetable. Do you have any experience with Apple? The fact that it is the plant's last output means that it includes seeds, which may be utilized to develop other apple trees. This is difficult to do with leaves, stalks, and roots.

7.6 Melon

Despite the fact that it is botanically a berry and hence classified as a vegetable, the melon is nevertheless referred to as a fruit due to the presence of seeds. Among the members of the Cucurbitaceae family is the melon, which is a very nutritious fruit that is high in water content, edible, and may help to hydrate your body.

It was discovered in Africa, Iran, and India and is easily distinguished by its vibrant colours, which include a greenish tint on the surface and a pink hue on the interior. Melon is a sweet fruit that is easily recognized by its vivid colours, which include a greenish tint on the surface and a pink hue on the interior. Antioxidants, which are good for human health, are also included in this category.

7.7 Okra

Because it includes seeds and develops from a flowering plant, however, okra is considered a fruit under the meaning of the term. It is possible to establish another okra plant from the seeds that have been collected. As a healthy fruit, it is high in vitamins C and A, and it may help with a variety of health problems, including diabetes, heart disease, and cancer cell growth. It may also help to reduce blood sugar levels in those who have diabetes. Despite the fact that okra is a vegetable that grows just once a year, its seeds lead many people to believe that it is a fruit.

7.8 Corn

The ovary of the corn plant, from which the seed develops, is often referred to as a fruit since it is the first stage of the maize plant's life cycle and contains the seed. Corn on the cob is a nutritious dried fruit that may be used in a number of pizza recipes. Thanks to the great grain in this meal, our empty tummies will be properly satisfied in no time. The term "caryopsis" refers to the whole seed coat of a corn plant, which protects the kernels from dust and other infections throughout their development. Corn seeds are what humans eat, and these seeds may be used to propagate new plants in the future if they are stored properly.

7.9 Avocados

A huge seed is covered by a layer known as the endocarp, which is then covered by the mesocarp (the fleshy edible component of the seed that you eat), and the exterior portion of the seed is known as the exocarp, which is removed by peeling. According to the USDA, avocados are true fruits, not vegetables. The enormous seed of academia is protected by three layers of protection. According to botany, the fruit is classed as a berry because of its large seed and is one of the fruits with just one seed, along with the mango. Avocado is a high-nutrient fruit that may be consumed by the majority of people in the United States, despite the fact that it is not very sweet. In the gym, your trainer might have told you to eat an avocado before going to work out if you eat vegan food in the morning.

7.10 Beans

Despite the fact that string beans seem to be vegetables, they are really fruits since they contain seeds that have the ability to re-sprout a new plant from the ground. It is now possible to find seeds for new blossoming bean plants in old string bean fruits that have dried up due to the maturation of the growing seed throughout the maturity process.

Throughout South Asia, string beans with immature seeds are a popular vegetable. Both vitamin K and calcium, both of which are abundant in string beans, contribute to the maintenance of a healthy bone structure. In addition, it contains vitamins A, C, and folic acid, as well as other minerals and antioxidants. Following a plethora of cooking demonstrations on YouTube, I discovered that it is wonderful and goes particularly well with potatoes. It's wonderful and filling at the same time.

7.11 Olives

Olives are a kind of fruit that grows on olive trees and are the size of little stones. They are harvested in the fall. The majority of people were unaware that it could be classified as a fruit, yet it is, along with dates, peaches, and other fruits. Due to the presence of seeds in olives, they are categorized as fruit rather than as a vegetable. In these fruits, you'll find plenty of vitamin E, which is beneficial to your skin. Antioxidants are also included since they are vital in the fight against free radicals and other harmful substances. It helps to enhance our immune systems as well as our physical appearance. Olives help to improve our levels of HDL cholesterol, which is good for our hearts.

7.12 Zucchini

Due to the fact that it originates from the flowers of a flowering plant known as a zucchini plant, zucchini is technically a fruit rather than a vegetable. Lots of water and nutrients are contained inside it. It is possible to create new plants from the seeds of an existing one. Hemp is a nutritious food that is high in skin-healing antioxidants such as vitamins E, C, and A. Consuming much zucchini has two advantages: it aids digestion and may reduce blood sugar levels. It has a high concentration of antioxidants, which helps to protect our cells from oxidative stress and degradation.

7.13 Apricots

Some of the health benefits of apricots include the prevention of anaemia, constipation, earaches, fevers, and skin disorders. In addition, apricots are beneficial to the heart, muscles, and wounds of the body. It is also believed to be healthy for the skin, which is why apricot is often used in cosmetic products. As an added benefit, apricots may lower cholesterol, protect vision against degeneration, aid in weight loss, strengthen bones, and maintain electrolyte equilibrium in the body. Apricots are botanically known as Prunus armónico, and they are little drupes that resemble peaches or plums in appearance and flavour. It is juicy and soft flesh that lies underneath the thin, outer skin. An apricot contains an inedible pit in the centre, which makes it potentially perilous to take the first major bite of it. They are often yellow or orange in colour, with a reddish tinge on one side of the flowering plant.

Given that it has been grown both in the wild and in ancient times, it is impossible to pinpoint the specific sequence of apricot cultivation across the world. Apricots are said to have originated in Armenia, which is where the scientific name "apricot" derives from. In addition to ancient Greece and Rome, numerous academics think that the earliest cultivation took place in India more than 3,000 years ago, according to archaeological evidence. The disputed origins of apricots are immaterial, but the health advantages they provide to humans are obvious. Whether you want to eat your apricots raw or dried, either option is appropriate.

Various applications include the preparation of jams, squashes, and jellies, as well as the preparation of other juices and syrups and the preservation of preserved fruits. Preparing and consuming apricots differs greatly from one culture to the next. For many years, they were a popular option for individuals seeking to enhance their health because of their unique, organic components, nutrients, vitamins, and minerals, which are all mentioned below. Apricot kernels may also be used to extract the oil from the fruit, which has a number of health benefits.

7.14 Bananas

A banana has twice the amount of carbohydrates, three times the amount of phosphorus, four times the amount of protein, five times the amount of vitamin A and iron, and double the amount of all other vitamins and minerals as an apple. Their natural sugars include sucrose, fructose, and glucose, among others. These carbohydrates provide the body with a rush of energy that lasts throughout the whole day almost immediately after ingestion.

According to research, two bananas provide adequate energy for a 90-minute workout. Sodium, which is rich in bananas, serves to keep the cardiovascular and nervous systems in good working order. Potassium, in addition to its role in muscular contraction, potassium also has a substantial influence on a wide variety of muscle-related functions, such as the maintenance of a regular heartbeat and the process of digesting. Several additional studies have linked low potassium intake to an increased risk of high blood pressure and stroke.

B6 is abundant in bananas, making them a particularly good source of vitamins. Among its many functions, this vitamin assists in the conversion of tryptophan (an amino acid present in protein) into serotonin, as well as the creation of haemoglobin, which is required for proper blood circulation. Vitamin B6 is necessary for the maintenance of a healthy immune system. Carbohydrates into glucose, which helps to maintain steady blood sugar levels.

7.15 Almonds

A quarter cup of almonds provides 70% of your daily vitamin E needs. Other nutrients found in these superfoods include magnesium, potassium, zinc, selenium, copper, phosphorus, biotin (vitamin A), riboflavin (vitamin B), iron, and fibre. Monounsaturated fat, which is an important nutrient, is also found in high amounts in these superfoods. Given that they have the highest concentration of calcium of any nut, they are the ideal nut for vegans who do not eat dairy products.

Aside from that, they contain amygdalin (commonly known as laetrile or vitamin B17), a controversial anti-cancer mineral that some believe may contribute to the body's ability to fight cancer. The phytosterols beta-sitosterol, stigmasterol, and campestral found in almonds have been shown to promote cardiovascular health. An almond serving per day may lower low-density lipoprotein (LDL) cholesterol, sometimes known as "bad" cholesterol, by as much as 10%.

However, it is not simply the fact that they lower cholesterol levels that makes them so helpful; their high quantity of monounsaturated fat makes them a vital component of many Mediterranean diets. A normal Mediterranean diet not only lowers the risk of heart disease and cancer but also increases the length of life of those who follow the diet. Include olive oil and even a glass of red wine in your Mediterranean-style diet as an easy way to include more nutritious foods into your daily regimen.

The Mediterranean diet is well-known for being low in saturated fat, high in monounsaturated fat, and high in dietary fibre. In a recent study including more than 1.5 million healthy adults, it was shown that following a Mediterranean diet is associated with reduced rates of cancer and cancer mortality, as well as decreased rates of Parkinson's and Alzheimer's disease. To follow the Mediterranean diet, you should get plenty of exercises, eat mostly plant-based foods such as fruits and vegetables, whole grains, legumes, and nuts, substitute healthy fats such as olive oil for butter, and season your food with fresh herbs and spices rather than salty seasonings, eat no more than a few servings of red meat per month, eat fish and poultry at least twice a week, and drink red wine only in moderation. The diet also highlights the importance of sharing a meal with family and friends, as well as the importance of gathering around a table with loved ones.

7.16 Grapes

When it comes to cardiovascular health, grapes are out of the norm. According to Romano, grapes have been linked to increased blood flow and lower blood pressure in studies through vasorelaxation. Grapes have been shown to be beneficial in lowering cholesterol, fighting inflammation, and assisting platelets in clumping. In their natural state, grapes have no saturated fat or cholesterol, and they are very low in sodium, making them a fantastic choice for a heart-healthy snack.

A recent study reveals that grapes may also be beneficial to the brain, in addition to their long-established heart-health benefits. In tests with older people with mild cognitive impairment, regular ingestion of grapes was shown to help preserve healthy metabolic activity in parts of the brain connected to early-stage Alzheimer's disease, when the metabolic decline begins to take hold.

A recent study discovered that people who consumed the most flavanols had a 48% lower risk of developing Alzheimer's disease; this is yet another reason to have more grapes. During a two-week pilot study in colon cancer patients, researchers discovered that daily ingestion of grapes decreased the expression of certain target genes associated with tumour formation. No harmful cells were affected by the grapes, which suggests that they could help keep the digestive system healthy.

7.17 Acorns

Some of the numerous health benefits of acorns include heart protection, increased energy, digestive help, and blood sugar management, to mention just a few. This nut is also beneficial for bone health, development, and repair. It also reduces inflammation, helps to avoid diarrhoea, and helps to improve the texture and look of one's skin. Acorns are produced by the Quercus and Lith carpus genera of trees, which are also known as oak nuts or acorns in other parts of the country. An external cupule, which is where the nut attaches to the oak branch, may be found on the nut's exterior shell and is responsible for its adhesion to the branch.

These nuts are between 1 and 6 centimetres long and 0.8 to 4 centimetres broad. They take between 6 and 24 months to mature and are available for harvest in the fall. During the winter months, the Northern Hemisphere's oak trees lose their nuts, which squirrels may collect for a winter food supply. Due to the fact that they were widely available and performed many of the same nutritional functions as grains, acorn nuts were a key food source for many early communities. Acorns, in fact, are still a frequent element in traditional Korean and Native American dishes today.

However, because of the tannins included in the uncooked acorn, it is not recommended to do so since it is difficult to digest. Boil or soak the acorns in water until they are no longer distasteful and the water is no longer brown. This is because of the high tannin content in these nuts, which may cause irritation to the lining of the stomach as well as other problems with your digestive system in other situations.

8

Chapter 8: The Healthiest Vegetables

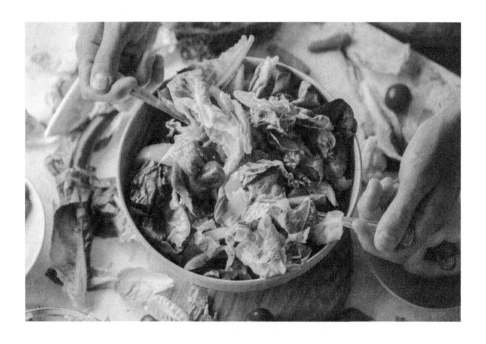

T rain harder, recover faster from activities and recover from injuries faster using a secret weapon that may also help to reduce inflammation in joints and enhance your energy levels, according to research. Something that your competitors aren't properly using. It's a great deal. It's right there in your kitchen. Green, white, yellow, orange, blue, and red is some of the colours available. In the first and most important instance, it is alive!

Vegetables serve as a connection between the dinner table and athletic performance. High-intensity workouts like sprinting, weightlifting, and plyometrics deplete the body's chemical fuel reserves; therefore, athletes must eat an increased number of fresh vegetables to make up for this depletion. Speed and power athletes may benefit from ingesting a broad range of veggies on a regular basis in order to get the most out of their central nervous systems. By focusing on your neurological system rather than your muscles, you may distinguish yourself from the rest of the pack and stand out from the crowd. When it comes to movement, the nervous system is in charge of determining how and when to do so. Win by providing nourishment to your neurological system. Animal protein and lipids are the primary sources of nutrition for the nervous system, and products make use of all of these nutrients.

When ingested alongside fresh vegetables, other nutrients are more readily absorbed by the body. Green leafy vegetables, which are an essential element of any athlete's protein-rich diet, aid in the activation of this enzyme. Even frequent eating of vegetable fibre aids in the absorption of the nutrients found in animal protein through the digestive system. Vegetables have a critical role in the intake of high-quality fats, which are required in the diets of athletes who perform at high speeds and with great strength. The lipids in vegetation aid in the digestion of the plant's roughage, which aids in the improved absorption of nutrients when fats are present in the diet. In this way, your insulin levels stay the same. This means that you can react quickly when you need insulin at the right time.

Opening bottles of drugs and taking what they believe to be vitamins and minerals are all part of an athlete's morning regimen. Despite the high cost of all of the bottles combined, a significant number of them wind up in the trash bin. It is possible to resolve the situation in an easy way. This is something our predecessors have been doing for at least a million years. Consume micronutrients derived from plants in their natural state. Folic acid pills (vitamin B-9) are superfluous when a simple salad may be served as a complete meal in its own right. Why consume vitamin C that has been synthesized in a laboratory when you can get your vitamin C from fresh produce? Your root vegetables should get their nourishment from the ground up.

A negative attitude toward vegetables is prevalent among the younger population in particular. Many individuals shun veggies due to the fact that they are not enjoyed by everyone. When it comes to vegetables, on the other hand, they should be highlighted as an essential part of maintaining a balanced diet. If a meal contains some vegetables, it is regarded as a well-balanced meal. The most nutritionally dense veggies are those that are picked fresh. This is the most effective method for ensuring that their taste and nutritional value are not compromised. Vegetables may be prepared and served in a number of different ways. They may be served with the main course or a side dish.

When it comes to preparing vegetables, there are a variety of methods available. Vegetables may be cooked, grilled, or deep-fried to your liking. When it comes to your health, each plan has its own set of advantages and disadvantages. Overcooking vegetables, in the view of nutritionists, is not a wise choice. More than 10 minutes of cooking time causes vegetables to lose a significant amount of their nutritious value. When this happened, the majority of the vegetable's nutrients were absorbed by the surrounding water. Fried vegetables, on the other hand, are not necessarily a healthy option. This is due to the fact that the oil in which the vegetables are cooked will cause them to get greasy. Finally, but certainly not least, dietitians recommend grilling vegetables. The reason for this is that grilling does not result in the loss of nutrients or exposure to excessive quantities of oil as other methods of preparation do.

In recent years, vegetables have emerged as a significant component of a nutritious diet, owing to the vitamins they provide. Plants have a lot of different nutrients, like potassium, vitamin A, vitamin E, vitamin C, folic acid (folate), potassium, and dietary fibre. The body reaps significant advantages from the consumption of these vitamins and minerals. Folate, for example, has been shown to increase red blood cell formation. Foods such as vegetables are a good source of dietary fibre, which has been shown to provide health advantages. It has been shown to lower cholesterol levels in the blood.

Having a high cholesterol level in the bloodstream may lead to a range of health problems, including heart disease. Fibre also has the benefit of assisting in the maintenance of normal gut function. Potassium is found in vegetables, and it is thought to help regulate blood pressure within a normal range. High blood pressure patients will benefit greatly from the consumption of vegetables. The antioxidant effects of vitamin A are beneficial to the skin. It makes the skin seem younger and more luminous when used regularly. Taking vitamin, A supplements may also help to increase one's visual acuity. The antioxidant effects of vitamin C are beneficial to the teeth and bones. Vitamin C also contributes to the absorption of iron as well as the healing of wounds, among other functions. Vitamin E, on the other hand, aids in the oxidation of important acids inside the cell.

It is also possible that eating veggies will lower your chances of acquiring diabetes and having a stroke. Additionally, some vegetables may be beneficial in the prevention of cancer, osteoporosis, heart disease, and kidney stones. It is also good to consume vegetables on a regular basis in order to assist with weight loss. A lot of this may be because the meals have a low-calorie density and much fibre in them.

8.1 Vegetables keep the vultures away

An athlete's performance suffers if they do not consume enough vegetables. It has the potential to cause subpar performance as well as muscle damage. Immune system deficiencies result in sickness and harm as a consequence of these deficiencies. The generation of free radicals that cause muscle damage is another side effect of intense exercise. Fresh vegetables include antioxidants that may aid in the fight against free radicals. The efficacy of antioxidants is increased when they are combined with plant nutrients (phytonutrients). In the end, this combination has a substantial influence on the outcome.

In recent studies, it has been shown that phytonutrients have a direct impact on the central nervous system (CNS). They are involved in cellular signalling, which has an impact on the way information is sent by the central nervous system (CNS). The anti-inflammatory qualities of this CNS message aid in the development and repair of the body's tissues. Speed and power athletes, who must train at a high level of intensity, are especially worried about the dreaded post-workout DOMS (discomfort of muscle after exercise) and DOMS (delayed onset of muscle soreness). DOMS may be controlled with the use of plant nutrients.

The ability to move fast and with great force. Athletes' pH balance is dependent on the consumption of fresh vegetables, which is why they should consume more of them. Getting to the bottom of this problem will be challenging. To achieve professional athletic status, anybody who does not have a God-given talent will have to put in endless hours of training and dedication. It is vital to continually strengthen the body in order to be able to apply more force to the ground. For athletes to keep up with their tough training and quick growth, they need a high protein intake in their diets.

So much protein combined with so much intense activity results in a significant shift in pH balance in favour of acidity. An acidic imbalance increases the likelihood of muscle irritation, soreness, and injury, all of which are undesirable. Furthermore, the acidic quality of the average American diet exacerbates the problem. Processed fats, such as those present in the majority of our processed foods, are acidic in the same way that the animal proteins they contain are acidic. Rice, coffee, and condiments are all high in acidity and should be avoided. When employing fruit concentrates and juices, it is vital to consider the acidity of the product. Because of our excessively acidic diet, millions of individuals suffer from stomach acid, and many blindly follow the multibillion-dollar pharmaceutical industry by purchasing "anti-acid" medications. Magic pills, on the other hand, are completely ineffective. With a healthy diet that includes plenty of fresh vegetables, you won't need to visit a doctor or take any additional medications to reduce acidity, injuries, or muscle soreness.

Changing an acidic pH balance to an alkaline pH balance demands ingesting a wide range of vegetables in order to be successful in this endeavour. Because hard exercise results in an acidic pH, athletes must consume a large number of vegetables in order to move the pH balance toward the alkaline side of the spectrum. There are a variety of additional options that may be beneficial. Wild honey has a high alkaline content. For athletes who train for speed, beta-alanine, an alkaline supplement, is a popular choice.

Green leafy vegetables, which are high in calcium and found in abundance in an alkaline diet, are also included in this diet. When a meal high in alkalinity is consumed rather than when calcium supplements are used while in an acidic environment, calcium absorption is enhanced. Calcium is vital for athletes that participate in high-intensity training, such as sprinters, since it helps to minimize inflammation and muscle soreness in the body. Green leafy vegetables, which contain calcium, may be beneficial in relieving painful joints after weightlifting. It increases the likelihood of catching a cold by strengthening the immune system.

In addition to the "internal broom" system, a diet rich in fresh vegetables are essential for proper digestion. When veggies are ingested on a regular basis, the fibre in them helps to sweep and clean the intestines. Better absorption is achieved as a consequence of increased nutritional contact with the gut surface. Interior surfaces continue to be stimulated, allowing them to digest food at a faster rate and with greater efficiency than previously. As a consequence, the body has access to a greater number of nutrients. When compared to whole wheat or oats, the fibre content of fresh vegetables is much greater.

No matter how much you like or despise vegetables, they are necessary for your overall health. Because you're already consuming them, the goal is to discover fresh and innovative ways to include even more of them in your diet. By following these easy principles, you may make it easier to eat more vegetables. The vegetables must be sliced into tiny pieces in order for this to be accomplished successfully.

Start your dinner with a simple green salad to set the tone. Start each evening with a huge salad before anything else is consumed during dinner time. Other vegetables should be used in the salad in addition to lettuce (the least nutritious green leafy vegetable). It doesn't matter what veggies you use; the most important thing is that they are fresh and vibrant in colour. Garnish your salad with olive oil, vinegar, and herbs dressing to get the most nutrition and flavour out of it. On other occasions, a Caesar salad or a Greek salad might be offered instead. You may also make a version of your favourite salad from Olive Garden. Dinner should include a salad, which should be regarded as obligatory.

Making a practice of eating a large bowl of vegetable-based soup on a daily basis can help you lose weight. Bones from chicken or ham may be used to flavour a big batch of homemade chicken soup. Experiment with a variety of soups, increasing the number of veggies in each one. The longer it stays in the oven, the better it tastes, and vice versa. Alternatively, leftovers may be frozen and consumed at a later date.

If you're already a ketchup consumer, there's no reason not to boost your consumption even more. Produce a variety of vegetable sauces and spread them liberally over your chips and meal. Use celery or carrot slices as a dipping sauce while you're preparing a meal for the family. To serve with tacos, make a large batch of salsa and guacamole from fresh avocados and set it aside. You can prepare a delectable vegetable sauce to serve on top of meat dishes in the same way you would ketchup. Another effective approach for getting liquefied vegetables is the use of juicers. Learning how to make vegetable juice with much pulp is a skill that can be taught. Even those who despise vegetables will be impressed by the flavour of this dish.

Eat your vegetables thinly sliced. Toss them in a cheese sauce or a butter sauce, or just bathe them in freshly squeezed lemon juice and serve as a side dish. It's usually a good idea to have a selection of fresh vegetables on hand for cooking purposes. The essential thing to remember is to make eating veggies a regular part of your routine.

As a last resort, go for organic products. When it comes to pesticides, many of the pesticides present in ordinary grocery store vegetables have a terrible effect on reactions, which is precisely what speed is built on. Pesticides, chemical fertilizers, and preservatives in concentrations as low as a few parts per million might cause nerve damage or dullness. It has been found that chlorpyrifos and dimethoate, two common commercial pesticides, can slow down and stop signals from the central nervous system (CNS) to muscles, especially fast-twitch muscles.

According to the Environmental Working Group, certain vegetables purchased at the grocery store contain considerable quantities of contaminants (EWG). In the produce area of your local grocery store, you may be able to locate a broad selection of dangerous commercial vegetables. Avocados, broccoli, cabbage, onions, and sweet peas, all of which can be bought in most shops, have earned the endorsement of the Environmental Working Group.

The great range of vegetables that may be found in our meals is one of the most significant components of our nutritional intake. Because of the high concentration of minerals and vitamins in them, they are crucial for maintaining general well-being. Vegetables provide vitamins, minerals, and other elements that assist in the creation of bones, teeth, and other structural components of the human body. Vitamins, minerals, and other nutrients contained in vegetables help the body function properly. Large intestine health is improved when vegetables have indigestible cellulose or roughage, which makes it easier to digest these foods.

Vegetable leaves are green due to the presence of chlorophyll II, a pigment that gives them their colour. Chlorophyll II is affected by the pH of the solution. When exposed to acidic conditions, it becomes olive green; when exposed to alkaline conditions, it turns dazzling green. The steam produced when vegetables are cooked, particularly when they are not covered, cause some of the acids to be released. Carotenoids, which are responsible for the yellow or orange colour of vegetables, are not changed by typical cooking techniques or pH changes.

Root vegetables are high in carbohydrates, which makes them a vital element of a balanced diet since they are the major source of nourishment. Green vegetables are most often consumed in the form of stews and soups made from them. Vegetables should be consumed as raw as feasible and as regularly as possible in order to get the maximum amount of nutrients. Bad cooking has the ability to cause considerable harm to a major portion of the values stored inside a structure.

When it comes to food preparation, herbaceous plants that are used as ingredients are often referred to as "vegetables." The taste and nutritional value of soups are enhanced by the addition of seasonings. The majority of their compositions are made up of pectic compounds, hemicelluloses, and cellulose, among other things. Vegetables include all of the nutrients listed above as well as many more. They also comprise water and mineral salts such as calcium, iron, sulfate, and potash, among other elements. It is dependent on the kind of green vegetable, as well as the quantity of roughage and water it contains, whether vitamins A, B and C are present in various quantities.

Fresh veggies include a high concentration of vitamins and minerals, making them a vital element of a balanced diet. The advantages of cellulose include the prevention of constipation as well as aiding digestion. Dyspepsia, on the other hand, is induced by vegetables that are old and gritty. Among mature, dry legumes, cow peas, soy beans, Bambara nuts, groundnuts, and all other beans and dry peas are rich in protein and thiamine content, as is the case with all other beans and dry peas. On the other hand, groundnuts are a particularly good source of the B vitamin niacin.

8.2 The advantages of consuming vegetables

There is a conspicuous gap in the debate about the health benefits of eating fruits and vegetables, even though women all over the world often encourage their children to do so. In many cases, vegetables are not very popular with youngsters, particularly when there are other alternatives available. This is especially true when there are other options available. However, wouldn't it be ideal if we could start developing good eating habits in our children from a young age by teaching them the value of vegetables and the benefits they can give from an early age? We should establish this thought in the minds of our adult selves and then pass it on to our offspring to continue the tradition.

8.3 Reasons why vegetables are beneficial to our health

Because vegetables provide a broad spectrum of vitamins and minerals that are not available in animal products, vegetables are essential to our health. Green vegetables are high in minerals such as iron, magnesium, calcium, sodium, and selenium, but yellow vegetables are high in vitamins such as vitamin A, vitamin C, B vitamins, and vitamin K. It is recommended that you consume at least two servings of a variety of vegetables each day in order to meet your daily nutritional requirements. Compared to any other kind of food, this is the most extensive type of food.

Another essential issue is what vegetables do not provide in terms of health benefits. Meat and carbohydrates are often criticized for having high fat and calorie content, which are attributed to a variety of health problems. As a result of the accumulation of plaque in the arteries, lipids and cholesterol are often blamed for the development of heart disease. Carbon dioxide (CO_2) and carbohydrates, on the other hand, have been linked to obesity and other health problems. This means you may consume as many vegetables as you like without putting your health at risk since they do not contain these harmful elements.

Another aspect contributing to the health benefits of vegetables is the presence of antioxidants in their composition. Antioxidants are very effective weapons in the fight against illness. Antioxidants are often used as disease-fighting agents, but they may also be used as analgesics to decrease the onset of pain and reduce inflammation in the body as well. Antioxidants, on the other hand, may help to enhance one's immunity.

Foods are rich in dietary fibre and aid in the removal of toxins and other waste products from the digestive system that has accumulated as a result of eating an unhealthy diet. Many digestive illnesses, as well as more serious issues such as colon and stomach cancer, may be alleviated as a consequence of this treatment strategy. In addition, having a healthy digestive system makes it easier to digest and absorb nutrients, which makes it easier to get the nutrients you need.

It is important not to underestimate the nutritional value of vegetables as a source of health benefits. These foods comprise both the beneficial nutrients you ingest and the harmful nutrients you avoid consuming in your diet. For starters, there are so many different types of vegetables available that you'll never run out of things to do with them. You may eat them raw, mix them into salads, or include them in your favourite dishes. Because there are so many different ways to include vegetables in your diet, it is simple to take advantage of the multiple health benefits that they may provide.

Despite the fact that there is a wide variety of alternatives available, everyone is aware that some meals are superior to others in terms of taste. Vegetables provide a vast range of vitamins, nutrients, and minerals, all of which are beneficial. Including vegetables in one's diet provides a number of health benefits. A few foods, including vegetables, have been shown to assist in weight reduction and the prevention of a variety of diseases, and they are among these foods. Many health benefits can be gained by eating vegetables every day.

These are just a few of the many benefits. In order to lose weight, you should increase your consumption of vegetables to the greatest extent possible. Unlike other "diet" meals, eating vegetables in their natural, unprocessed state contains no fat, unlike other "diet" meals. People may eat as many vegetables as they want without worrying about packing on the pounds since vegetables are low in saturated fat. Aside from that, many vegetables are high in fibre, which may help individuals feel satiated for longer periods of time after eating them. Consequently, consumption will be lower as a result of the impression of being full. People who are trying to lose weight may want to eat more vegetables because they give their bodies more energy.

One of the various benefits of eating vegetables is that they help to keep you healthy and prevent illness. According to the World Health Organization, vegetables include vitamins, minerals, and phytonutrients that may help prevent a variety of ailments, including heart disease and cancer. It has been shown that antioxidants contained in many vegetables help to reduce the number of free radicals in the human body. People who eat vegetables on a daily basis have been shown to have a decreased risk of developing certain health concerns. If you want to stay healthy, you should eat at least five servings of fruits and vegetables every day.

Aside from fruits and vegetables, vegetables are one of the few foods that have been scientifically shown to have a beneficial effect on health. Some people augment their vitamin and mineral intake with supplements, although vegetables are a wonderful source of these elements in large quantities. People's health advantages of increasing their vegetable consumption are many. Vegetables help to increase energy levels while also improving the look and texture of the skin, making them a vital element of any nutritious diet. A range of cooking methods is available to enhance the nutritional content of vegetables for customers. When compared to their non-vegetarian counterparts, vegetarians are often healthier.

As people get older, their vision is more likely to suffer as well. By consuming a range of fruits and vegetables, one may improve one's eye health in a number of different ways. According to research, some phytochemicals contained in a range of vegetables may reduce the chance of developing eye degeneration. Lutein, a pigment present in spinach and other leafy greens that may help protect against eye diseases such as cataracts and macular degeneration, has been shown to be beneficial. In the past, vitamin A has been known as a powerful antioxidant and eye-protective compound. Carrots have a lot of vitamin A in them.

Despite the fact that there is a wide variety of alternatives available, everyone is aware that some meals are superior to others in terms of taste. Vegetables provide a vast range of vitamins, nutrients, and minerals, all of which are beneficial. Including vegetables in one's diet provides a number of health benefits. A few foods, including vegetables, have been shown to assist in weight reduction and the prevention of a variety of diseases, and they are among these foods. Many health benefits can be gained by eating vegetables every day. These are just a few of the many benefits.

In order to lose weight, you should increase your consumption of vegetables to the greatest extent possible. Unlike other "diet" meals, eating vegetables in their natural, unprocessed state contains no fat, unlike other "diet" meals. People may eat as many vegetables as they want without worrying about packing on the pounds since vegetables are low in saturated fat. Aside from that, many vegetables are high in fibre, which may help individuals feel satiated for longer periods of time after eating them. Consequently, consumption will be lower as a result of the impression of being full. People who are trying to lose weight may want to eat more vegetables because they give their bodies more energy.

One of the various benefits of eating vegetables is that they help to keep you healthy and prevent illness. According to the World Health Organization, vegetables include vitamins, minerals, and phytonutrients that may help prevent a variety of ailments, including heart disease and cancer. It has been shown that antioxidants contained in many vegetables help to reduce the number of free radicals in the human body. People who eat vegetables on a daily basis have been shown to have a decreased risk of developing certain health concerns. If you want to stay healthy, you should eat at least five servings of fruits and vegetables every day.

Aside from fruits and vegetables, vegetables are one of the few foods that have been scientifically shown to have a beneficial effect on health. Some people augment their vitamin and mineral intake with supplements, although vegetables are a wonderful source of these elements in large quantities. People's health advantages of increasing their vegetable consumption are many. Vegetables help to increase energy levels while also improving the look and texture of the skin, making them a vital element of any nutritious diet. A range of cooking methods is available to enhance the nutritional content of vegetables for customers. When compared to their non-vegetarian counterparts, vegetarians are often healthier.

As people get older, their vision is more likely to suffer as well. By consuming a range of fruits and vegetables, one may improve one's eye health in a number of different ways. According to research, some phytochemicals contained in a range of vegetables may reduce the chance of developing eye degeneration. Lutein, a pigment present in spinach and other leafy greens that may help protect against eye diseases such as cataracts and macular degeneration, has been shown to be beneficial. Carrots have a high concentration of vitamin A, which is considered to protect against cataracts and blindness.

8.4 Vegetables help you to live longer and healthier

Until recently, the term "organic" had not yet made its way into our everyday vocabulary. It wasn't all that long ago that the word "hippie" was used to refer to someone who was active in the counterculture movement. My family and I made the commitment five years ago to consume organic foods in our diet solely. When I was younger, my family and friends thought it was strange and unnecessary for me to go to such lengths. A buddy dubbed me a "hippy chick" because of the organic lifestyle that my family and I follow.

Organic food is now widely available. It has only recently become popular for people to notice the benefits of doing so, notably the benefits of eating organic vegetables. Much dispute exists when it comes to the differences between organic and conventionally grown food. The vast majority of organizations and scholars will assert that there is no differentiation between the two. There will, however, be an equal number of those who believe that there is a difference. The objective is to complete your research and make a conclusion thereafter.

As a result of my own study, cancer patients are often advised by their doctors to adopt an organic diet and way of life. As a result, I think organic food has certain scientifically proven health benefits to provide. The Food and Drug Administration has acknowledged that pesticides are present at small levels in the food we eat. The decision on what is proper in their view, on the other hand, is up to them. The FDA inspects a staggering number of compounds, which is a testament to its effectiveness. If just a small percentage of our food is tested by the FDA, how can we know what is in the other 95%?

Organic farming is successful, and this is a proven truth. The chemicals that are now being used are completely unnecessary. Organic vegetables offer several benefits, and we should make use of them. Then, what exactly are the benefits of consuming organically cultivated produce? Let's look into it a little further.

Organically grown vegetables offer a higher concentration of nutrients than conventionally grown vegetables. The majority of conventional vegetables are grown using chemical fertilizers, which stimulate growth by flooding the crop with water. Conventional vegetables, on the other hand, are typically composed primarily of water. The amount of minerals available has steadily decreased over the last six decades. Since then, we've started pre-picking crops, started using chemicals to keep them fresher for longer periods of time, and overprocessed the food in our warehouses and distribution centres, among other things.

Another benefit is that pesticide residues are less likely to be ingested. According to scientific evidence, pesticide residue has been demonstrated to produce a variety of symptoms, including headaches, tremors, sadness, anxiety, and a lack of energy, among others. Even if the vegetables are rinsed, the residue remains on their vegetables. Additional specialists are concerned about the influence of various pesticide residues on the same meal, which is a concern shared by numerous others. Is the combination of these substances harmful to our health?

Children are especially sensitive to the effects of pesticide residues since their organs are still developing at the time of exposure. According to certain studies, toxic exposure has been related to developmental abnormalities in both children and adults. In addition, you are protecting your children, which is another reason to use this solution, as we said before.

Take into account the environmental impact as well. Organic farming provides environmental advantages that exceed the expenses. Increased effectiveness, improved soil structure, and water conservation are all benefits of using this method. Organic fruit is still up for debate, but there is much evidence that organic vegetables are better for you.

The simplest and most effective technique for improving your health is to consume more vegetables in their natural state. A diet high in green vegetables may help protect you against a variety of maladies, including heart disease and cancer, as well as skin conditions. That's not all, however. It may also have the additional benefit of slowing the ageing process in your body. If you follow these easy cooking guidelines, you will be able to get the numerous health benefits of leafy green veggies.

In addition to being low in fat and calories, green vegetables are rich in fibre and low in fat and calories. Furthermore, fibre is an essential weight-loss element since it lowers your appetite while simultaneously filling your stomach. All of the nutrients found in leafy green vegetables, such as folic acid, magnesium, potassium, and a wide range of phytochemicals, are beneficial to your heart health. These foods can help people with type 2 diabetes because they have much magnesium and aren't very high in sugar.

8.5 Maintaining bone health by eating green vegetables

Folate, a vitamin K-rich substance found in leafy greens, is essential in the synthesis of osteocalcin, a protein that is fundamental to bone health. Folate is present in leafy greens in high concentrations.

- Pasta, broccoli, and spring onions are just a few of the numerous green leafy vegetables that are high in iron and calcium that can be found.

- Everyone should be aware of the fact that fresh green vegetables are rich in vitamin A, which is a vitamin helpful to the eyes, and that everyone should eat more fresh green vegetables as a result. Antioxidants such as zeaxanthin, vitamin C, and lutein may all be beneficial in preventing eye damage. Macular degeneration and cataracts are two conditions that affect the eyes.
- They contain water, which helps to keep you hydrated while also improving the look of your skin.
- Beta carotene, which is present in leafy green vegetables, is a carotenoid that assists in the repair and development of tissue.
- There are many folates in these meals, which is an important ingredient for the body's production of serotonin. Serotonin, on the other hand, is a mood-enhancing chemical.
- There are several health benefits to eating green vegetables. Nevertheless, there are certain disadvantages to doing so that should not be overlooked. If you take a lot of blood thinners or other medicines on a regular basis, talk to your doctor before eating dark green vegetables.

Vegetables are sometimes seen as a necessary evil that must be endured rather than as a wonderful delicacy to be enjoyed. Because the concept of "eating our peas" brings up images of a dreaded activity, it's easy to see how the phrase has been entrenched in our collective consciousness. As you know, fruits and vegetables are full of nutrients, and for a good reason as well.

Increasingly, the United States and UK government suggests that we fill half of our plates with these healthy meals at each meal. Fruits and vegetables do not earn points in popular diet programs such as Weight Watchers, making them a fantastic option since they are guilt-free and packed with nutrients at the same time.

There is a large list of health advantages associated with vegetables and fruits that dietitians are well-versed in. These foods have high quantities of vitamins, minerals, fibre, and antioxidants, all of which are beneficial to the body.

People who eat these foods may be less likely to get diabetes, high blood pressure, heart disease, and cancer.

According to the Centers for Disease Control and Prevention, more than nine out of ten Americans eat fewer nutritious fruits and veggies than the daily recommended serving size of 2 to 612 cups. The average individual consumes approximately a cup of vegetables and one piece of fruit on a daily basis. Consuming a plate of fruits and vegetables is astonishingly simple when compared to other food groups. One serving of vegetables is half a cup of cooked vegetables or a cup of raw fruits and vegetables.

8.6 Nutrition Facts

- Calcium is a mineral that is important for bone and tooth health, as well as for muscle function.
- Folate decreases a woman's chances of having a child who is born with congenital disabilities.
- Iron is a nutrient that is necessary for the correct functioning of cells and the bloodstream.
- Magnesium is also important for healthy bone growth and the normal functioning of enzymes in the body, which helps to avoid muscle cramps and high blood pressure, among other things.
- Potassium is essential for maintaining a normal blood pressure level.
- Vitamin A is important for good eyesight and skin, as well as for protecting your body from getting sick.
- Vitamin C assists in the healing process and improves the health of the teeth and gums. Vitamin C is an antioxidant.
- The antioxidants in fruits and vegetables, as well as pigment-enhancing micronutrients like those found in fruits and vegetables, may help protect against a wide range of diseases and other conditions.
- Fibre makes you feel full, but it also has a lot of other health benefits, like lowering cholesterol and keeping blood sugar levels stable.

- Even if you make a concerted effort to include more fruits and vegetables in your diet, you may find it challenging to eat enough of them. According to the experts, grated carrots or shredded zucchini may be used in a variety of baked goods, such as muffins or pancakes. It is possible to get the benefits of the vegetable without actually eating it.

Make sure to chop your fruits and veggies into bite-sized pieces so that you always have something to snack on. Make a veggie tray that you can snack on anytime you want, and use your imagination to put it together. It is possible to eat vegetables in a number of ways, all of which are helpful to your health in one way or another. Can food be often more cost-effective and easily available throughout the year, despite the fact that fresh or frozen produce contains a few more nutrients than tinned food does?

8.7 Vegetables for losing weight

When looking for the best veggies for weight loss, the majority of individuals are looking for a list of the healthiest vegetables to consume in order to lose weight. Find out what they are by going through the whole book. Reduce your calorie intake in order to get a thinner and more toned look, and the best vegetables for weight loss make it easier to achieve this goal with ease. Low-calorie diets are now widely regarded as a weight-loss method since they help to lower the amount of fat that is stored in the body's fat cells.

As an example, prior research has shown that leafy green vegetables are beneficial in the control of both appetite and obesity. Leafy plants are likely to be high in both water and fibre content. So, they make a great addition to any weight-loss plan, and even more so if they're used with a weight-loss pill or other supplements. Furthermore, not only does this improve the results of weight loss, but it also helps to improve digestion and the metabolic process overall.

Eating more green veggies may have a positive impact on one's overall well-being. Which green leafy vegetables are the best when it comes to reducing weight? Many individuals like the variety of green leafy vegetables that are available. Following the recommendations of various health experts, including green vegetables in your meals and dishes may help you lose weight quickly and easily. They usually say that patients should eat seven or more servings of leafy greens each day in order to get the best results.

Some people may be uninterested in a list of the best leafy greens for weight loss, while others may find it useful. Others are opposed to leafy greens, and some even gag at the thought of consuming them. Occasionally, an allergic response to certain green vegetables might occur, and it is important to get medical advice before consuming these vegetables in large quantities. If you want to keep your health, you should eat a variety of leafy green vegetables, like kale or collard greens, every day.

In addition to being high in fibre and pectin, apples are also high in antioxidants. Pectin is a fibre that stops the body from absorbing extra fat and also helps to lessen hunger. Because of the high-water content, it is possible that a significant amount of poison will be washed out. Consuming celery's skin in its whole, which includes a considerable quantity of fibre, is highly recommended. Grapefruits, on the other hand, have been shown to aid with weight loss. According to the new research, compounds present in leafy greens reduce blood insulin levels by acting on the body's own systems. As a metabolic process enhancer, it assists in weight reduction and fat burning by increasing the rate at which fat is burned.

9

Chapter 9: Powerful Healthy Superfoods

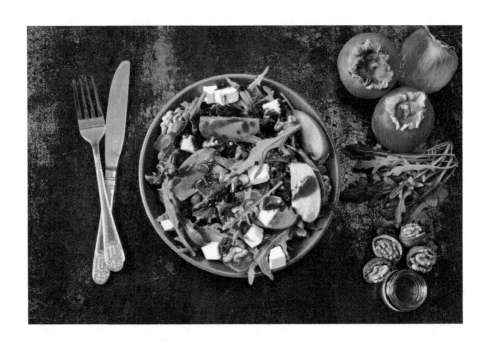

S uperfoods include a wide range of nutrients, including vitamins, minerals, and antioxidants. As a general rule, they are best taken raw or lightly cooked in order to retain their nutritional value as much as possible. Fruits and vegetables such as apples and berries, as well as vegetables such as broccoli and cauliflower, fall under this category. In the next section, you will find a list of superfoods, as well as information on what nutrients they contain and what possible health advantages they may have to offer. Whether you're trying to recover from an illness or just want to maintain a healthy diet, this advice will be of assistance. Despite hearing the term "superfoods," have you ever wondered, "What exactly are superfoods?" "Have you ever asked yourself, "What exactly are superfoods?" We'll take a look at what they are and how they could be of value to you since many people are talking about them.

When we say "superfoods," we are referring to foods that provide considerable health advantages, mostly as a consequence of substances produced by plants in their preparation. These substances are referred to as phytonutrients in the scientific community. People who eat certain foods may benefit their bodies in a positive way, and doing so puts them on the right path to a healthy future. When it comes to "superfoods," blueberries are a good example, and their health advantages are well-known.

Blueberries are not only sweet, but they are also an excellent source of phytonutrients, which are essential for optimum health. If you were to look into blueberries, you would find that they include a variety of important nutrients, such as Vitamin C, Manganese, dietary fibre, and others. In the same way that many other superfoods do, blueberries are high in antioxidants and may help you battle the effects of ageing, heart disease, and other common health issues. They also include anthocyanins, which have been shown in tests to be beneficial in the fight against cancer because of their blue colour.

Just by looking at one individual superfood, you can get a good idea of how these foods may be able to assist you in being healthier. In the produce section of your local supermarket, you'll find the vast majority of the superfoods

you're searching for. The absence of phytonutrients in the produce section is due to the fact that they are obtained from plants. If you want to get the most nutrients out of your meals, you should always choose the freshest options available. When it comes to frozen blueberries, for example, they do not provide the same nutritional value as fresh blueberries would.

Superfoods may be found in a variety of places other than the fruit department. Fatty fish, such as salmon and tuna, contain omega-3 fatty acids as well as other health-promoting components. Another example is the use of soy-based goods. There is a range of phytonutrients found in soy-based milk and cheeses that are not found in normal dairy products, including vitamin E. The items are also fortified with the vitamins and minerals that you would normally get from traditional meals, ensuring that you are still obtaining food that is fortified with the nutrients your body needs.

9.1 Superfoods are the healthiest foods you can consume

It is a kind of food that is high in nutrients, such as vitamins and minerals, as well as micro-and macronutrients, that is referred to as a "superfood." They're jam-packed with everything the body needs to be healthy and fight sickness as well as the ravages of time and the elements. They certainly are. One may choose and select from a wide array of superfoods. Incorporating superfoods into your diet has a number of health benefits, and this chapter will go over a few of the more noteworthy of these benefits, as well as how to go about incorporating them into your diet.

It was dieticians and nutritionists who first developed the word "superfood" to refer to foods that are rich in nutritional or therapeutic value. Many people are beginning to see that their health issues may be traced back to the processed foods they eat, which are often rich in sugar, high fructose corn syrup, and salt. They are also beginning to recognize that food is nature's medicine. A variety of superfoods have been shown to be effective in the treatment of inflammatory diseases such as rheumatoid arthritis and heart disease, as well as the prevention of the building of dangerous cholesterol in the body. In the next few paragraphs, we'll talk more in-depth about foods like these and why they're so good for you.

Originally from Central and South America, avocados are now grown all over the world in tropical locations, with the majority of production occurring in the United States. It is green, egg-shaped, or pear-shaped, and somewhat larger than an apple, with a large pit in the centre. The darker the skin of the fruit, the riper it is. This superfood contains 75 per cent of its calories from heart-healthy monounsaturated fats; it also has 60 per cent more potassium than a standard banana, as well as high levels of vitamins B, E, and Avocados are abundant in dietary fibre, which is another advantage of consuming them regularly.

Avocado eating has been shown to reduce blood cholesterol levels when there is a surplus of fruit. According to one study, those who ate avocados for just seven days had a significant 22 per cent drop in their harmful cholesterol levels.

Ordinary potatoes have been shown to be detrimental to human health, but sweet potatoes, which are basically a root and very distantly related to regular potatoes, are far healthier. Sweet potatoes are high in complex carbohydrates, dietary fibre, vitamins B, C, and beta-carotene, as well as beta-carotene, all of which are beneficial to the body. Apart from their great nutritional content, sweet potatoes are considered superfoods because they are abundant in complex carbs, as we previously described in this book. When a person consumes meals that are rich in simple carbohydrates, insulin levels increase, stimulating the body to produce and retain more body fat. When it comes to gaining weight, this is one of the most prevalent factors to take into consideration. People who eat sweet potatoes and other superfoods that have complex carbs might be able to eat many carbs without gaining weight.

Other natural superfoods, in addition to acai, goji, mulberry, and other tropical fruits, include broccoli, eggs, fresh spinach, wheat and barley grass, raw cacao, salmon, olive oil, spirulina, and chia seeds, to name a few. There is a vast selection of these items that include vitamins and minerals that help your body stay strong and healthy, fend against illness and disease, and keep you looking younger. This isn't the only reason why you should include these foods in your diet. There's no difference between seeking a boost in energy, libido, or antioxidants and looking for them. It is advised that you search out the specific superfoods that will assist you in achieving your own health goals as described above. In any case, the best method to improve your overall health is to take a broad range of superfoods on a regular basis.

Follow the perimeter aisles of supermarkets, where all of the fresh produce is kept, in order to guarantee that you are consuming superfoods that are high in nutritional value. Visit farmers' markets and health food stores, where you'll discover a diverse selection of superfoods as well as knowledgeable staff who can answer your questions about nutrition.

9.2 The advantages of consuming superfoods

It is possible to have several motivations for including superfoods in your diet, but each of them is based on the premise that you should eat for your health rather than for convenience. In the first place, you must be motivated to learn more about the foods you consume and how they affect your overall well-being. When a health concern arises, it is common for people to turn their attention to their nutritional habits as a result.

The obesity epidemic in this nation is reported extensively in the news on a daily basis by the media. As the number of people who have diabetes, heart disease, and cancer continues to rise, the quality of their meals will be called into question. In our country, there is a large number of people who eat meals that are out of balance, low in nutrients, and not intended to promote good health. The most often marketed food alternatives are those that are convenient, flavorful, and that encourage highly processed industrial meals that are rich in fat and sugar.

Fast food, ready meals, salty snacks, processed foods, and sugary cereals are all promoted in ways that have a direct influence on the diets of hundreds of thousands of people. Convenience is emphasized in food advertisements as a selling factor. People are encouraged to eat a high-calorie, low-nutrient diet by appealing to their sense of beauty rather than their ability to think logically.

When I'm at the grocery store, I'm often taken aback by what I see in people's grocery carts. Along with the sugary drinks, salty snacks and cereals, frozen pizza and prepared meals, the cart is stuffed to the brim with groceries. Nothing new has been added to the shopping cart.

Without making an effort to educate themselves on the nutritional value of the items in their shopping carts, obesity and bad health will be the inevitable result for many people. Increased obesity rates among youngsters who eat much fast food and who are fed this kind of diet on a regular basis will be shown. It is also possible that these children's eating habits will carry over into adulthood, even as they develop.

In the case of superfoods, if a person isn't interested in them because they lack the will to eat healthily, they will not be interested in them. One of the most significant benefits of consuming foods from the list of superfoods is that they help you lose weight. "Superfoods" are foods that are high in minerals and vitamins yet low in calories, hence earning the name. A nutrient-dense, calorie-restricted diet is required for successful weight reduction efforts. When it comes to losing weight, it's best to eat foods that have the most nutrients per calorie that you eat.

Superfoods may be used to gradually lower your calorie consumption by gradually substituting high-calorie, low-nutrient meals with healthier alternatives. According to an ancient wives' tale, habits are established after

28 days of repeating the same thing over and over again until it becomes automatic. Your efforts and patience will be required if you want to train yourself to develop new eating habits successfully. When you've been eating the same way for a long period of time, it might be difficult to break the habit. Having realistic goals and planning for them together has a better chance of working out.

It is necessary to begin by gradually decreasing the quantity of sugar in your diet. It's important to keep track of what you eat and how much you consume at each meal if you want to improve your diet. The first step is to consult with your physician. The ability to exert control over one's diet and food choices may be one of the primary reasons why many people want to lose weight. For those of you who have been diagnosed with diabetes or who are at risk of acquiring type II diabetes, your doctor should have urged you to lose weight and keep track of what you eat.

Unfortunately, many doctors are more concerned with prescribing medications than they are with encouraging a healthy diet. In my opinion, continuing to eat in the same manner as you did before to develop diabetes and then taking drugs to manage the condition is the wrong course of action. Patients, doctors, dietitians, and former patients are among those who have successfully cured type II diabetes by dietary changes. A diet high in superfoods may help you maintain or improve your immune system.

Nutrition, devotion, and a healthy diet that emphasizes foods that are high in nutrients, low in sugar, or otherwise too processed are the most important parts of a healthy diet. These are the things that make a healthy diet.

Therefore, include superfoods in your daily diet on a regular basis. You may design your diet around the following basic list of superfoods, which you can get at your local health food store: If you want to strengthen your immune system and stay healthy, the superfoods on the following list are a wonderful place to start.

- There are many different types of green leafy vegetables.
- Legumes are available in a variety of kinds.
- Various types of potatoes
- Cruciferous plants are those that contain cruciferous elements.
- There is a large selection of berries available.
- Seeds and nuts are a kind of food.
- Coconuts

9.3 Use superfoods to lose weight and have a long life

The superfoods for weight loss are also beneficial for your general health. As you include these nutrients into your diet and remove junk food and fast food, you will see a transformation in your body. You may consume large quantities of these foods to aid in the regularity of your bowel movements and the cleansing of your colon. Ideally, you should go to the restroom twice each day at the very least. If you aren't exercising, it is possible that constipation and old faecal matter have accumulated in your body. By cleaning out your colon with superfoods and colon cleansing procedures, you may be able to lose pounds of fat and get rid of a bloated stomach.

Instead of quick oatmeal, choose steel-cut or whole oats, which are higher in fibre and contain more nutrients. A healthy breakfast choice, oatmeal provides omega-3 fatty acids, folate, and potassium and is an excellent source of fibre. Additionally, this high-fibre superfood may aid in the reduction of LDL (bad) cholesterol levels as well as the maintenance of healthy arteries. Fruit may be added to sweeten it, or rosemary and sea salt can be sprinkled on top for a more rustic look and feel.

Avocados will increase your consumption of heart-healthy fats if you include them in your diet. Avocados are a fantastic source of monounsaturated fat, which may help lower LDL (bad cholesterol) and enhance HDL (good cholesterol) (good fat). Avocados are also a terrific addition to salad dressings and sauces. Adding avocado to a kale salad is a simple way to boost the nutritional value of the dish while also adding taste.

The superfood known as Popeye's spinach may help you lose weight because it is high in lutein, which is an antioxidant; folate, which is a B vitamin; potassium, which is a mineral that is present in high amounts in the human body; and fibre (another type of antioxidant). If you eat many vegetables, this is a surefire way to improve your digestion and overall health.

Add a sprinkle of ground flaxseed to your oatmeal or whole-grain cereal to get the most out of your daily intake of fibre, omega-3 and omega-6 fatty acids, and other nutrients. Additionally, it may be blended into smoothies or salads and consumed in this manner.

Blueberries, raspberries, strawberries, and blackberries are all high in fibre and antioxidants, and they are also delicious. In a recent study, it has been shown that blueberry-rich meals help rats lose weight while also improving their general health, including lower cholesterol levels and improved glucose control.

Soy. It's no surprise that soy is a staple in the diets of many vegans and vegetarians, as well as many others. Soy milk, when combined with oatmeal or whole-grain cereal, is a filling and filling supplement that keeps you satisfied for a long period of time. To save money and time, opt for unsweetened soy milk and sweeten it with honey or agave nectar at home whenever possible.

Water. While water is not considered a food by most people, it is very important for both your health and weight loss. You'll find that when you're dehydrated, your liver needs to work more to maintain water balance in your body than it does to aid in fat burning.

Keep your body hydrated by drinking plenty of water throughout the day. It is important to drink enough water to keep your stomach satisfied and to remove toxins from your system. It doesn't matter if you wake up hungry in the middle of the night or not; drink some water to check whether dehydration is the cause.

Legumes rank ninth on the list of superfoods for weight loss. Legumes, lentils, and chickpeas are all rich in dietary fibre, as are black and kidney beans. These heart-healthy snacks are high in omega-3 fatty acids, calcium, and soluble fibre. They are also low in saturated fat.

Psyllium, The use of psyllium will help you go to the toilet even if you're the most constipated person in the world. To begin, take a tablespoon in the morning with two full glasses of water during the first several weeks of treatment. It may be necessary to add a second tablespoon of butter to your evening meal if the first doesn't work. Remember to drink plenty of water when taking psyllium since it will transform into a gelatinous material in your body if you don't. It is possible to get constipation because your body is not receiving enough psyllium water.

Only because Acai berries are so excellent at aiding in weight loss does this fruit have its own category within the fruit world. A recent popular trend in the health food industry is the use of acai berries, which originate in South America and have a high concentration of antioxidants and other minerals. It has been linked to a variety of benefits, including weight loss, improved skin, a stronger immune system, a greater feeling of well-being, and more.

9.4 Mood-boosting foods

The majority of people are aware that eating a nutritious diet is the most effective way to maintain good health. Vegetables and lean meats are essential components of a balanced diet, but junk food is detrimental. The majority of people are not aware that there are such things as "superfoods," yet there are some foods that may qualify as such. The nutrients included in superfoods are crucial for maintaining a healthy body and mind, as well as for weight loss. They are high in nutrients, such as vitamins, minerals, and antioxidants, all of which may be beneficial in cancer prevention.

Not only are these superfoods beneficial to your health, but they are also delicious. Superfoods come in a variety of flavours and textures that will please even the most discriminating eaters, despite the fact that not everyone has the same palate for food. At the very least, one of these superfoods should be a regular component of your diet. Better yet, establish a target for a small number of people. When it comes to getting the most out of a superfood, a little goes a long way, so keep that in mind.

We've collected a brief list of superfoods to help you on your journey to a happier and healthier life. Read on for more information. The following is a healthy diet recommendation for today: Consume at least one serving of each of the following superfoods per day:

9.5 Almonds

Almonds are high in iron and magnesium, and they are also naturally low in saturated fat, which makes them a healthy snack option. Any diet may benefit from the addition of unsalted almonds, which are both delicious and healthy. Almonds are a terrific snack to consume in order to help people lose weight or maintain weight. They are also an extremely effective appetite suppressant.

9.6 Avocados

Avocados have a plethora of nutrients, including high concentrations of vitamins A, B, C, D, E, and K in a single serving, as well as fibre and potassium. Avocados are a terrific source of healthy fats, which our bodies need in order to function properly. Because they are so easy to cook, vegetables like this one make an excellent complement to any supper. Acai avocados are also a great source of folate, which is important for the growth of healthy tissue.

9.7 Blueberries

Antioxidants and vitamins found in microscopic blueberries not only assist your mind and body but also aid in your overall health by strengthening your immune system and keeping you healthy. Regarding the quantity of fibre that they contain, blueberries are no different from other berries in this respect. Fresh blueberries may be added to oatmeal or yoghurt, or they can be blended with other ingredients to make a wonderful and refreshing fruit smoothie that can be served for breakfast, lunch, or dessert. Your mind and body will be thankful to you for the rest of the day.

9.8 Broccoli

Because of its abundant supply of vitamin D, broccoli is considered a superfood. Vitamin D may be found in a variety of foods, and the sun is a good source of vitamin. Additionally, consuming half a cup of broccoli three times a week may aid in the development of strong bones and the maintenance of a healthy weight, in addition to benefiting your respiratory and digestive systems. Broccoli is delicious whether it is cooked or raw, steamed or fried, or baked. Drizzle on a little extra virgin olive oil when cooking or baking to get an additional dose of superfood deliciousness.

Dark chocolate contains antioxidants that assist the body in its fight against cancer. A half bar (of a full-size candy bar) has 200 calories, 10 grams of sugar, and 20 grams of fat, making it a treat that should be enjoyed in moderation at all times.

9.9 Extra-virgin olive oil

Olive oil, on the other hand, is a fat-free product. This kind of fat, on the other hand, is very beneficial to your cardiovascular system. Because a teaspoon has just 60 calories and contains 7 grams of fat, it will only contribute 60 calories to your daily caloric intake. Make your own salad dressing with olive oil and serve it as a condiment with your meals. Even if you are not aware of it, extra virgin olive oil is beneficial to your cardiovascular health, which is fantastic for everyone.

9.10 Honey

The high concentration of vitamins and minerals in honey, despite the fact that it is mostly composed of water, natural sugars, and sucrose, makes it an ideal alternative to sugar, high fructose corn syrup, and artificial sweeteners. Honey contains a number of minerals, including pollen, calcium, zinc, and vitamin B6, in addition to pollen, calcium, zinc, and vitamin B6. Honey may be used to enhance the flavour of drinks and meals. In addition to being a great superfood, it also helps wounds heal and prevents infections.

9.11 Kale

If you tune in to any cooking show these days, you'll notice that kale is a popular ingredient to use. Kale may be the newest superfood trend, but there's a solid reason for it to be so popular. Consuming kale may help to decrease cholesterol levels in a natural way. Eating kale, which is tasty and packed with nutrients that might help you accomplish exactly that, may help you significantly cut your risk of developing a variety of cancers, including prostate cancer.

Eat lean meat to ensure that your body gets the protein it needs while avoiding excessive fat. The amino acids present in lean cuts of beef, chicken, and turkey are critical for the formation and maintenance of lean muscle tissue. If you have to eat meat every day, try to eat leaner cuts of meat in smaller amounts.

9.12 Pistachios

Mixed nuts are another excellent source of protein. As a side benefit of consuming a small handful of mixed nuts for your mid-morning or mid-afternoon snack, you will be less likely to consume junk food that is detrimental to your health.

As an alternative to reaching for chips or crackers when you're craving something crunchy, try frying up some broccoli or kale with your favourite spices to give it the zing you want. Do you have a sweet tooth that is begging to be satisfied? It is possible to squash such urges with a little bit of dark chocolate, a cup of hot tea with honey, or a plate of blueberries drizzled with honey.

When you include these superfoods in your diet, you'll feel like a whole different person. If you have more energy to go out and about, you'll become fitter, stronger, and healthier than you've ever been before. The state of your health determines your level of happiness, and the state of your health determines your level of contentment. It's difficult to conceive of a more compelling reason to include these superfoods in your diet. I really hope that these diet suggestions will assist you in beginning your journey toward a better life

Chapter 10: Benefits of Meats, Seafood & Grains

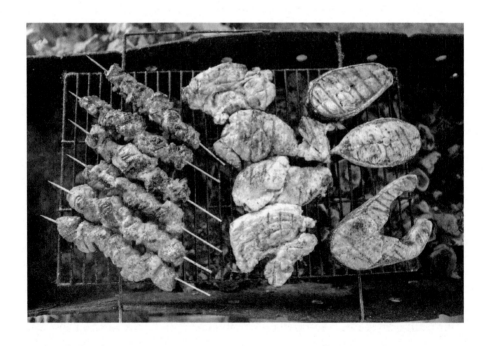

W hen it came to buying beef, things used to be a whole lot simpler
back then. The development of new labelling words and claims,

on the other hand, has resulted in a rise in consumer complexity as a consequence of a large number of new labelling terms and claims available. Even though it may seem daunting at first, accurate and genuine information about an animal's existence, encompassing the whole of its life cycle, is helpful to both the animal and the person who purchases the product. Simply said, when an animal is cared for and allowed to express its natural behaviours in a manner that enables it to reach its full potential, the meat, flavour, and nutrition of the animal are all more likely to be of higher quality and so more desirable to the client.

The ideal situation would be for animals to be able to graze on open pastures all year long, allowing them to ingest a variety of nutritious and fibre-rich plants, such as perennial and annual grasses, broadleaves, legumes, and a variety of seasonally available species of plants. Animals may be given supplemental dry hay or fermented crops (also known as silage, haylage, or bale age) to supplement their diets when they are not in season, providing them with delicious, nutritious, and easy-to-digest animal feed. A diverse diet, such as that eaten by animals in the wild or those raised on diversified small farms that were popular throughout history until World War II, contains the majority of the fat found in their bodies. Polyunsaturated and monounsaturated fats are the most common types of fat found in the bodies of animals. The omega-3 to omega-6 fatty acid ratios in grass-fed beef are higher than in conventional cattle.

Evidence suggests that consuming grass-fed beef decreases the risk of heart attack, stroke, and other inflammatory conditions such as arthritis and arthritis-related thrombosis as well as arrhythmia because of the meat's greater omega-3 fatty acid content. However, further research is needed to confirm this. Chickens and other birds that are allowed to roam and peck outdoors in vegetation in search of bugs, worms, and other small creatures have a higher omega-3 fatty acid ratio than those kept inside. Given the abundance of linoleic acid in pasture grasses, meat from grass-fed ruminant animals (such as cattle and sheep) is likewise higher in conjugated fatty acids than meat from grain-fed ruminant animals (such as deer and elk) (CLAs). Contrary to popular belief, CLA is a generic term that refers to a variety of distinct forms of linoleic acid, each of which has been demonstrated to provide health benefits, such as lowering or suppressing the effects of cancer-causing chemicals, despite containing trans fats. CLAs provide many of the same health benefits as omega-3 fatty acids, including the ability to reduce inflammation.

There were a variety of causes that influenced farmers' decisions to abandon natural, grass-fed agricultural systems during the course of the preceding century. The feeding of grain to animals in CAFOs (concentrated animal feeding operations, often known as feedlots or CAFOs) in the late nineteenth century was shown to create more palatable, soft meat marbled with fat while simultaneously increasing the quantity of saturated fat in the meat. A growing number of widely used techniques have arisen, all with the objective of transforming animal husbandry into an industrialized industry that is both large-scale and cost-effective. Bovine spongiform encephalopathy (BSE), sometimes known as mad cow disease, was first seen in the United Kingdom in 1976. It was caused by the practice of adding cheap animal by-products from ruminant animals to animal feed, which spread the disease.

Another example is the extensive use of antibiotics in animal feed, which is becoming more common. Pigs and poultry have both been subjected to industrialization attempts that are comparable. Despite the fact that the animals have been developed for certain characteristics that benefit the consumer, they have suffered from painful physical or unusual behavioural repercussions as a result of their breeding. When larger pigs began biting the tails of smaller pigs, many farmers believed they had "solved" the issue and shaved the tails off the rest of the pigs to make them seem smaller. The bones of poultry that have been bred to have more breast meat may become overwhelmed as a consequence of the increased weight placed on them during breeding. Because of the focus on lowering production costs, it is hard for hens and pigs to exhibit their usual behaviours in crowded and dismal living conditions. This has a negative influence on the animals' physical and emotional well-being.

Seafood is one of the few dishes that really defines "global" eating since it helps us to get an understanding of various cultures via our culinary experiences. At our local markets, you may get wild Alaskan salmon and sablefish, farmed Norwegian salmon and Scottish sockeye, Mexican sardines, British Columbian halibut, South African hake, scallops, prawns, and a variety of other fresh seafood items. And the list goes on and on.

However, despite the fact that seafood is one of the easiest proteins to prepare, many individuals are more apprehensive about making it at home than they are about eating it in a restaurant setting. For the most part, it comes down to adapting cooking techniques to suit the fish or seafood you're using and keeping things simple. The flavours of the accompanying sauces and side dishes should complement rather than overpower the flavour of the fish. As much as seafood's great taste and ability to be used in a wide range of dishes have undoubtedly made it so popular, the nutritional benefits of cold-water fish, especially fatty varieties, have long been known as a major source of the heart-healthy omega-3 fatty acids.

10.1 Seafood provides a variety of health benefits

- The essential oils present in seafood are critical to maintaining a balanced diet. Additionally, oils are wonderful flavour enhancers in addition to supplying us with the fuel we need to run our vehicles. In addition, they are a significant source of fatty acids, which are beneficial.
- The unique qualities of seafood oils have a significant positive impact on our health. The polyunsaturated fatty acids eicosatetraenoic acid (EPA) and docosahexaenoic acid (DHA) present in this oil are two of the omega-3 polyunsaturated fatty acids (DHA).
- Given that our bodies are only capable of producing a small number of

these essential fatty acids on their own, we must get them from external sources. One of the most effective methods to get these vitamins and minerals is through the consumption of seafood. Oil is the second most commonly used ingredient in seafood.

- If you consume seafood once or twice a week, it may have beneficial effects on your health. Fresh fish, which contains these essential oils, may be acquired by consumption. It is also possible to obtain supplements that include oils derived from seafood.

- It is possible that oils produced from fish might help prevent some of today's most serious ailments, such as Alzheimer's disease and asthma. These oils include fatty acids such as omega-3 and omega-6.

- Omega-3 fatty acids have been shown to lower blood pressure and improve the symptoms of rheumatoid arthritis. As well as this, they assist in the development of an infant's brain and eyes.

- The omega-3 fatty acids present in seafood may help to prevent osteoporosis. The oils play a role in this because they help our bodies absorb calcium more effectively, which helps to protect our bones from becoming brittle over time.

- According to current studies, omega-3 fatty acids also help to strengthen people's immune systems, thereby reducing their chance of contracting an illness.

- Foods high in omega-3 fatty acids have been shown to reduce blood pressure, making them especially advantageous for those who suffer from high blood pressure.

- Seafood also includes omega-6 fatty acids, which are beneficial in addition to omega-3 fatty acids. This method has the potential to contribute significantly to human growth and well-being.

- Consuming seafood is a great strategy to lose weight and keep it off. For decades, seafood has been a mainstay of many weight-loss diets across the world. When compared to diet medications, seafood is an excellent natural source of nutrients that are beneficial to people.

- Frozen fish, on the other hand, has a tendency to deteriorate extremely quickly. As a consequence, you should begin preparing it as soon as possible after receiving it. Here are some suggestions for preparing seafood:

- If you aren't planning on preparing the seafood soon, you should store it in the freezer for no more than two days at the most.
- Thaw the fish in the refrigerator or, if required, in a bowl of cold water. Keep it away from direct sunlight and heat sources if at all possible. This is due to the possibility that the nutritional content of the seafood would diminish.
- Wonderful seafood recipes may be used to create a variety of scrumptious fish dishes. Seafood may be prepared either grilled or fried. By including fruits and vegetables in it, you may make it even more delicious and nutritious. You may marinate the meat to get rid of the odour while also improving the flavour.
- A fear of choking on the small bones found in shellfish has led some people to refrain from eating them altogether. If you need help getting these fish bones out, you can ask the fish store for help.
- Consider the potential health benefits of eating seafood in addition to the delicious flavour it provides.
- If you have a liking for seafood, you should get acquainted with nutrition science.

In spite of the fact that the present health and diet situation in the United States is not optimum (or is it because of this?), more individuals are paying attention to nutritional science now than at any other point in human history. As "information age" citizens, we have unprecedented access to knowledge, and we can learn a great deal about how to eat a nutritious diet and get the advantages of doing so. Nutritional sciences are one of the most fascinating and rapidly expanding academic fields available, and the rate at which new discoveries are being made will astound even the most seasoned academic. Aside from that, it seems that as the number of dietitians in general increases, it appears that more and more of them are falling in love with Alaska seafood. In fact, the nutritional data on Alaskan seafood is so convincing that you don't have to be a genius to see that increasing your consumption of this kind of seafood will have a significant beneficial influence on your physical and mental well-being.

The truth is that the more you learn about Alaska's seafood nutritional data, the more you'll want a delicious wild Alaska salmon fillet, some enormous and soft King crab legs, or any other exquisite and enticing specimen of seafood obtained from the coastal waters of Alaska! Many people have focused more on the hazards of mercury and PCBs in fish than on the health benefits of eating seafood in general, despite the fact that seafood has long been recognized to be a rich source of nutritionally beneficial compounds. However, despite the fact that these chemicals have been identified at harmful levels in particular regional harvests across the vast Alaskan coastal fishing waters, the specimens gathered each year show minimal to non-existent quantities of these compounds in their composition. To be more specific, the clean and bountiful marine ecosystems of the North Pacific are some of the world's last remaining sources of the best seafood on the planet.

The much-maligned Omega-3 and Omega-6 fats are unavoidable when considering Alaskan seafood nutrition, as is the case with all seafood. It doesn't matter which omega fatty acid you choose to concentrate on; omega fatty acids have been shown to benefit cholesterol levels, cardiovascular health, eye health, and even brain health. It's as simple as that: Alaska seafood is your ticket to a long and prosperous future.

10.2 The nutritional benefits of eating meat

Despite the growing popularity of vegetarianism, meat continues to be an important element of a well-rounded nutritional plan. A lot of people's diets include vegetables and fruits since they are considered to be more nutritional alternatives to meat. However, this is not the case in this instance. Meat has a diverse spectrum of nutrients that are not found in other dietary types.

Eating meat may help to enhance your metabolism while also providing you with the energy boost you need. Several health benefits of meat-eating are listed below. These are some of the benefits of meat consumption:

10.3 Sources for superior protein

Eating meat is a convenient way to get a significant amount of high-quality protein. Protein supplies us with energy and aids in the maintenance of the health of our muscles and organs, among other things. A full source of nutrition, animal protein contains all of the amino acids necessary for human bodies, making it a complete protein supply. However, it is possible for the body to manufacture certain amino acids. However, some amino acids must be acquired from animal proteins. Combining multiple different kinds of plant sources may result in a complete protein supply, but this requires careful consideration and may be difficult to achieve. Eating red meat is a simple way to make sure your body gets the amino acids it needs on a regular basis.

10.4 Minerals

Zinc, iron, and selenium are just a few of the minerals that may be found in animal products. The iron content of red meat is much greater than the iron content of plant-based diets. Haemoglobin is used in the production of haemoglobin, which is responsible for transporting oxygen throughout the body. It is possible that an iron deficit may result in anaemia and other health concerns. Zinc is a critical mineral for the maintenance of healthy hair, skin, and nails. Zinc may be found in abundance in red meat.

This disorder may be caused by a zinc deficiency, which may cause a decrease in one's sense of hunger. Growing evidence suggests that increasing the quantity of red meat ingested by children may improve zinc deficiency. Selenium may also be contained in animal products such as meat. Taken in the form of supplements, selenium may help your body break down fat and other organic substances more quickly.

10.5 Vitamins are abundant in this food

Meat has a high concentration of vitamins. Vitamins play an important role in the wellness of your body. Meat is a good source of vitamins A, B, and D, among other nutrients. All of these vitamins may be found in abundance in meat. These vitamins are also good for the health of your central nervous system and your mental health, as well.

10.6 Fat

Contrary to common belief, a balanced diet necessitates a reasonable quantity of fat intake on a daily basis. You need fat in your body in order to develop your brain and to be able to tolerate unpleasant events in your environment. Among the facts contained in beef are linoleic acid and palmitoleic acid, which are both fatty acids. These types of fat help to keep your body healthy by preventing it from cancer and infections that may be harmful.

Meat consumption offers a host of health benefits. Meat contains a variety of nutrients, including protein, minerals, vitamins, and fats. These kinds of nutritional benefits are very difficult to come across in a substitute. Increase the strength of your body and the quality of your health by eating meat on a regular basis. General health will improve, and you will be less susceptible to infections and viruses as a result of these changes. Consuming two to three meat meals every week will provide you with all of the benefits listed above, as well as make you feel great.

10.7 The health advantages of grains

What do you think about some rice or couscous? This is a question that is often asked in my home. Many others, on the other hand, feel that rice is the only grain that may be consumed. Only when you've experimented with a diverse selection of grains from across the world will the question of which grain to utilize for a meal become clear. It's possible that a certain kind of rice, such as Bhutanese red rice, would provide the remedy, but we've been exploring the universe of complete foods for decades. Quinoa, Kamet, millet, and farro are some of the other grains that may be used as substitutes. It might be bulgur, spelt, wild rice, or barley blended with rye, or it could be something else entirely. It is possible that corn could be on the menu for my wife, and steel-cut oats will be on the menu for me.

Traditional grains are becoming increasingly popular among health-conscious consumers as a result of the numerous nutritional benefits they provide. Consequently, grains have been raised from poor food to a diet that is almost revered. Quinoa, for example, appears on restaurant menus as often as it does in the recipe sections of newspapers. When it comes to making a final selection of grains, flavour and texture are the most important considerations.

For those with busy schedules, some grains may be cooked in under 30 minutes, making them an excellent alternative for people on the go. "Whole grain" is a term that is used to describe a kind of grain in meals. For the simple reason that they are what they are: whole grains. Whole grains include all of the nutrients present in the seeds of cereal grass plants. When the seed is sprouted, the grain becomes a rich and compact source of nutrition for humans as well as for other animals. Buckwheat and quinoa, for example, are really seeds from plants that are not cereal grasses but rather legumes and hence are not considered grains.

As a consequence, they are classified as grains for the most prevalent of these reasons: they are functionally and nutritionally equivalent to cereal grains in terms of nutrition and function. The three basic structural components of whole grain are the bran, the germ, and the endosperm, which are all found in equal amounts. B vitamins, trace minerals, and lignans, which are potent antioxidants, may all be found in the bran, which is the grain's outer layer that contains the greatest amount of fibre. Bran acts as a barrier between the contents of the seed and the germination process. Humans may also benefit from it because it helps to keep the nutritional value and nutritional quality of whole grains intact during storage. The germ is the seed's life force; it is the component of the seed that sprouts and develops into a new plant after being planted.

Vitamin E, trace minerals, and unsaturated fats, as well as B vitamins, minerals, and protein, are present in high concentrations in the sprout's initial few days of growth, as are other essential nutrients. A small amount of starch, protein and trace amounts of vitamins and minerals are retained in the seed's endosperm, which serves as fuel for the sprouted grain throughout its early developmental stages. The fact is that you're not alone; if you've ever wondered why you should incorporate whole grains into your diet. The combination of nutrients found in these foods—fibre, vitamins, minerals, and phytonutrients—may help decrease cholesterol and stabilize blood sugar levels, as well as reduce the risk of heart disease, diabetes, and various malignancies.

There is some evidence to support this claim. Consuming whole grains may also help to lower the chance of developing diabetes, obesity, and heart disease. To get the most nutritional value out of your food, choose whole grains that still have their seeds attached. All whole grain goods are made from grains that have been handled in a way that preserves the majority of all of the fundamental components (bran, germ, and endosperm). Grains that have been cracked, crushed, flaked, extruded (like pasta), or somewhat pearled are included in this category (removing only a tough, inedible outer hull). Grain products that have been processed to remove the bran and germ, mostly preserving the starchy endosperm, are known as refined grains (and refined carbs).

Important phytonutrients such as dietary fibre, vitamins, minerals, and antioxidants, as well as lignans, phytosterols, and a plethora of other plant compounds, such as are lost as a result of the refining process. In the past, it was difficult and costly to refine wheat, and as a result, white flour was reserved for the rich and powerful. While the Industrial Revolution was taking place, white bread became more affordable as a result of new technology making it more cost-effective to manufacture white flour. Because of their reputation as a symbol of wealth and luxury, they continued to be regarded with high respect for a long period of time after their death. Refined grain products are popular for a number of reasons, one of which is that they are more lucrative for producers than unrefined grain products. Whole grain products have a shorter shelf life than refined grain products because the germ contains more oils that might become rancid.

10.8 Bran

Bran contains phytic acid, which may form bonds with minerals and prevent them from being absorbed by the body. At least one nutritional advantage may be derived through refining: People who don't receive enough minerals in their diets or who consume much bran are more likely to suffer from this problem. In comparison to processed grains, whole grains provide far higher health benefits. Several flour companies add nutrients back into their products to make up for the nutrients that are lost during the milling and processing process.

As a consequence, this is not a panacea for all problems. As a general rule, only five of the essential vitamins and minerals are provided, resulting in refined grains being deficient in a wide variety of essential elements and dietary fibre. In terms of nutrition and flavour, there is little question that whole grains are better and that they should be the primary focus of your diet on a regular basis, if not entirely. Many individuals find them to be a fresh and exciting experience. When it comes to supplying whole grains, time is often stated as a justification for skipping them in the meal plan. Including more whole grains in your diet is a very straightforward process that takes little time.

The best time to start is with breakfast. This is partly due to the fact that we like to eat more nutritious grains at this time of day. An old-fashioned favourite, oatmeal has long been recognized as the best way to ensure a consistent supply of energy throughout the day. Even if you have a busy schedule, you can whip up a tasty hot cereal from any sort of whole grain, possibly topped with some fresh or dried fruit, in no time at all. If it is prepared properly, there is no need to cook any kind of rolled, cracked, or finely ground grain for more than twenty minutes. A slow cooker may also be used to cook entire grains over an extended period of time.

The best dry ready-to-eat cereals include shredded whole grain cereals, muesli, granola made without oil, and low-fat granola that is very moderately sweetened, among other things. As a side dish for lunch and dinner, grain may be served with stir-fried or grilled vegetables. As a side dish with beans, tempeh, pork, or chicken, or as a basis for soups and stews, grains are a versatile ingredient. They're a terrific starting point for casseroles, croquettes, salads, and stuffing, among other dishes. Sprinkled on top of soups, they may also be used as a thickening agent to add texture and body to the dish.

11

Chapter 11: Develop Healthy Eating Habits

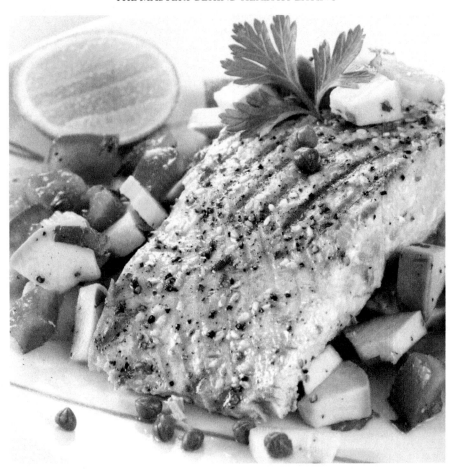

A healthy and active lifestyle may enable you to be more productive in both your business and personal lives if you follow it consistently. Your ability to do more tasks will increase since you will not get fatigued as rapidly as you would otherwise be. As a side benefit, you may have more confidence in your way of life now that you've built up a robust immune system via regular exercise and eating a nutritious diet. Many individuals find it difficult to keep track of their food consumption on a daily basis because it takes too much time. The facts you uncover, on the other hand, will almost certainly take you by surprise.

When you include the little candy bar and the two cookies, you come up with a grand total of Every day, we do activities that have a significant influence on our nutritional intake, but we don't pay attention to them since they are routine. The most effective method of establishing a healthy eating habit is to consume more fruits and vegetables than we would normally consume each day. Despite this, why do we continue to purchase potato chips at the grocery store rather than fresh fruits and vegetables?

All of this boils down to one thing: consuming junk food enhances our desire for more of the same in the future. Have you ever questioned why you would consume something as small and inconsequential as a beverage? Does it seem like it would be possible to consume the whole box of Cheez-crackers in one sitting? After tasting something for the first time, your body responds by prompting you to consume more of that particular food item. Having the ability to train yourself to live a healthy lifestyle and consume red grapes on a regular basis will help you achieve your objectives. Despite the fact that it will be challenging, success is not impossible. If you follow these five steps, you will be able to train your brain to make healthier snack choices in the future.

If you want to lose weight, you must understand the most effective techniques to improve your diet and exercise habits. It is possible that participating in these activities may assist you in developing techniques that require dedication and extraordinary management abilities. It's good to have good habits like eating a well-balanced diet and exercising every day.

11.1 Evaluate your physical condition

Begin by becoming familiar with your own physical body. In kilos, how many pounds do you weigh in pounds? What's the present status of my lungs in this situation? The following are some of the questions you should be asking yourself: Do you have any particular goals in mind while you're writing this?

There are a variety of fitness tests that you may do at your local clinic to get a better understanding of the state of your body.

After a period of getting to know one's physical self, achieving a goal becomes a lot more straightforward. If you are overweight or obese and wish to lose weight, a well-balanced diet and weight-loss program should be considered. When the time comes, you may realize that this practice has provided you with significant benefits.

11.2 Dietary supplementation

When you've gotten a better grasp of your body's nutritional requirements, it's critical to establish a regular eating regimen. It is recommended by physicians to use the standard food pyramid as a guideline for estimating how much food you may consume in a particular amount of time.

You are consuming a diet that is high in protein and carbohydrates will allow your body to operate efficiently. In certain circles, macronutrients are referred to as proteins and carbohydrates, respectively. You will lose strength because you don't get enough vitamins and minerals.

Protein-rich meals, such as meat and poultry, are required for the growth and development of a healthy adult body. Sugar and bread may provide you with the energy you need to get through the day, but they should be avoided at all costs. In addition to vitamins and minerals, fibre, and other dietary supplements, there are many other types of dietary supplements that should be taken. When you have a diet plan in place, it is simple to meet your daily calorie requirements while still maintaining a nutritious diet.

11.3 Regular physical exercise

They contend that maintaining a healthy weight range is essential for living a healthy lifestyle. This does not rule out the possibility that you are correct in your assumption, but it does not imply that you should engage in strenuous physical exercise. If you want to get your heart rate up in the morning, you may go for a jog first thing in the morning. The benefits of exercising include keeping your body and mind in optimum shape, as well as keeping your intellect sharp.

When you are physically active, your body may be better able to deal with stress, and it may even speed up the process. In the long run, this may assist the body in producing more protective hormones, which is advantageous. As a result, your ability to respond quickly to normal situations and make better decisions will get better. This is because your mind will be more alert because it will be more alert.

You should do some exercise straight away after your fitness evaluation in order to get the best outcomes possible. You don't want to be in a situation with someone who is about to go off the rails. It's probable that you'll feel physically and mentally exhausted at some point. Any time you start a new exercise plan, you should talk to your doctor or a fitness expert.

Maintaining a nutritious diet and engaging in regular physical activity are the only ways to create a healthy lifestyle. By making smart food and exercise choices that take into account all of the many factors that play a role in these decisions, you will be able to improve your health and well-being in the long run.

11.4 Learn how to build healthy eating

In accordance with the consensus of health care professionals, maintaining healthy eating habits may have a positive impact on your overall health. As a result, in addition to assisting you in losing weight, healthy eating programs may also assist you in improving your overall health and well-being. One of the most important parts of healthy eating is avoiding overindulgence in fast food and preparing meals on a regular basis. When it comes to losing weight, people need to understand that fad diets and restrictive eating are not the solution, and they should avoid them at all costs.

Because they will gain back many more pounds than they lost when they are hungry, despite the fact that they may lose a few pounds while fasting, they should avoid doing so. Weight loss training regimens that are both quick and effective, as well as healthy food programs, are recommended in order to obtain the desired body shape and tone. Whenever you embark on a new endeavour, be certain that you are committed to seeing it through. Only then will you be able to get the required results.

Here are a few suggestions to get you started: Instead of eating two or three substantial meals throughout the day, you may want to consider eating 4-6 small meals throughout the day. Rather than consuming a wider range of high-carbohydrate and high-fat foods when you divide your meals into smaller amounts, opt for a greater choice of healthy fruits and vegetables. Chew each mouthful carefully and completely to ensure that you get the most nutrients possible from your diet. As a result, experts believe that people who properly chew their food are more likely to eat fewer overall because they are more likely to feel the fullness of their stomachs sooner. It's also a good idea to stop eating when your stomach sends a signal to your brain that it's full. When you're attempting to lose weight rapidly via exercise, you should never skip breakfast.

Skipping breakfast increases your chances of overindulging in the hours that follow, which will contribute to your total weight gain. Consequently, it is imperative that you avoid skipping breakfast at all times. Aside from eating a diet rich in fruits and vegetables, you should consider having other healthy meals such as lean meat to round out your nutritional intake. It is critical that sugar intake be carefully managed and kept to a minimum to the greatest extent feasible. Participating in a weight-loss fitness program may assist you in losing weight more rapidly. Whether you're looking for a weight-loss training program or a healthy diet and exercise plan, choose the best person to help you.

"How can I lose weight fast and effectively?" is a question that many people who wish to lose weight quickly ask themselves. It is unlikely that we will ever have to be concerned about our weight if we do not find ourselves in a situation where we will be unable to escape the criticism that comes with it. There is a multitude of reasons why we would want to lose weight quickly, such as preparing for an impending event or for another compelling purpose. In order to be successful with this quick weight loss strategy, you must first prepare yourself properly. When it comes to weight-loss programs, setting them up is usually easy, but keeping them going for a long time can be hard.

If you want to see any program through to completion, you must put up your best effort and remain committed to it throughout. First and foremost, you must have a clear awareness of what is going on within your body and how you want to adjust it in order to create good changes to your health. According to the American Heart Association, moderate movement every day for seven days a week for at least six weeks will help you lose weight rapidly and safely. It is essential that this training routine be combined with the appropriate calorie intake in order to be successful. If you follow this diet religiously, you can expect to lose 5 pounds in the first week.

Cardiovascular exercise is the most efficient form of weight loss, but it may be complemented with other activities such as strength training to get greater results. If you want to burn more calories with a simple workout, you must have a greater amount of muscle mass. Reduce your carbohydrate intake while increasing your physical activity and lowering your calorie intake at the same time. According to the American Heart Association, food high in starch encourages fluid retention and, if consumed in large quantities, may have a substantial role in the development of the syndrome. It is also recommended that you avoid foods that are high in carbs, sugars, and animal fat, in addition to those that include meat and dairy products. All of these items may be replaced with healthier options such as fruits and vegetables, soy products, seafood, low-fat dairy products, and lean meats. It follows that increasing your protein intake will aid your weight-loss efforts. It is also critical to maintain a record of your progress and accomplishments as an added bonus.

Exercise and eating the recommended meals should be done with a journal to keep track of your progress. If you follow these instructions, you will be able to sustain your enthusiasm throughout the remainder of the time. Maintaining an activity journal is the most efficient way to do this. This journal, which you should keep in a safe place, may be useful in helping you keep track of your progress and events as they occur. You may use this chart to track your progress toward your weight-loss goals and to identify when you need to put in additional effort to achieve your objectives.

12

Chapter 12 - Conclusion

I t is possible that the route to a healthy diet will appear different for each individual depending on their current state of health, diet, and manner of living. Please let us know how much you enjoyed our book on the nutritional importance of fruits, vegetables, seafood, and whole-grain items in your diet. We're here to tell you that eating a diet high in vegetables, fruits, seafood, and whole grains is beneficial to your health in the long run.

Many vegetables are really rich with nutrients that are essential to your overall health and well-being, so eat up! It is our hope that the information in this book will help you make healthy eating a part of your daily life and reap the benefits!

13

References

- Healing Spices, edited by B. B. Aggarwal and D. Yost, was published by Sterling Publishing Company in New York in 2011 and is available online.
- J. Burg et al. (2008). Motivation, talents, and environmental opportunity are all factors that influence healthy eating. Family Practice is a kind of medical practice that focuses on the care of the whole family.
- K. R. Camargo et al. (2013). Medicalization, pharmaceuticalization, and health imperialism are among the terms that come to mind. the Department of Public Health and Welfare, number 29 (5)
- Cullen, K., Thompson, D., Boushey, C., Kennelman, K., Chen, T.-A. Cullen, K., Thompson, D., Boushey, C., Kennelman, K., Chen, T.-A. (2013). Teen Choice: Food and Fitness is a web-based program that promotes healthy food and physical exercise for teens. The program is being evaluated. Health Education and Promotion Research
- S. Deshpande, M. Basil, and D. Basil have collaborated on this project (2009). An adaptation of the health belief model is used to examine the factors that influence healthy eating habits among college students. Health Marketing Quarterly is published quarterly.

- Aminopterin, K.; Goatee, C.; Kaczmarski, P.; Janssen, I.; Janssen, I.; Dawson, M.; Aminopterin, K.; Bartley, N. (2012). Obesity maps in Canada are being updated to reflect the current state of the disease. The Canadian Journal of Public Health is a journal that publishes research on public health in Canada.
- Hausman et al. (2012). Hedonistic logic is used in the selection of healthy food intake options via muddling-through. The Journal of Business Research is a scholarly publication dedicated to the study of business.
- Melanin, J., Heasman, M., and Heasman, M. (2001). Part 1: The Functional Foods Revolution: Will Healthy People Lead to Healthy Profits? Part 2: Routledge Publishing Group, New York, NY. S. Innis, E. Baglo, and A. Cardinal collaborated on this project (1999). Aspects of food product creation and usage that go beyond implementation include the involvement of doctors, healthcare professionals, and consumers. The European Journal of Clinical Nutrition is a peer-reviewed journal that publishes research on clinical nutrition.
- M. Katan and N. Ros have published a paper in which they argue that (2004). The promise and the pitfalls of functional meals. Critical Reviews in Food Science and Nutrition is a journal that publishes critical reviews in food science and nutrition.
- S. Levy, S. B. Fein, and M. Stephenson have published a paper in Science (1993). The amount of nutrition knowledge on dietary fats and cholesterol varied from 1983 to 1988. The Journal of Nutrition Education is a peer-reviewed journal that publishes original research on nutrition education.
- Reduced to a single word: Lowry et al. Galuska et al. Fulton et al. Wechsler et al. Kan et al. Collins et al (2000). Physical exercise, diet selection, and weight control are all important objectives and practices for college students in the United States. Preventive Medicine: An American Journal of Preventive Medicine,
- N. Michelada, G. Christodoulides, and K. Tor ova are among those who have contributed to this work (2012). Motivations and obstacles to healthy eating: A cross-national examination of the factors that influence

them. International Journal of Consumer Studies is a peer-reviewed journal that publishes original research on consumer behavior.

Printed in Great Britain
by Amazon

83606622R00078